OXFORD PAIN MANAGEMENT LIBRARY

Chronic Pain

Edited by

Andrew Dickman MSc MRPharms

Senior Clinical Pharmacist,
Marie Curie Palliative Care Institute,
Liverpool, and the Cardiothoracic Centre,
Liverpool, UK

and

Karen Simpson FRCA

Consultant in Pain Medicine and Senior Lecturer,
Leeds Teaching Hospitals Trust,
Seacroft Hospital,
Leeds, UK

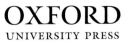

OXFORD
UNIVERSITY PRESS

OXFORD
UNIVERSITY PRESS

Great Clarendon Street, Oxford OX2 6DP

Oxford University Press is a department of the University of Oxford.
It furthers the University's objective of excellence in research, scholarship,
and education by publishing worldwide in

Oxford New York

Auckland Cape Town Dar es Salaam Hong Kong Karachi
Kuala Lumpur Madrid Melbourne Mexico City Nairobi
New Delhi Shanghai Taipei Toronto

With offices in

Argentina Austria Brazil Chile Czech Republic France Greece
Guatemala Hungary Italy Japan Poland Portugal Singapore
South Korea Switzerland Thailand Turkey Ukraine Vietnam

Oxford is a registered trade mark of Oxford University Press
in the UK and in certain other countries

Published in the United States
by Oxford University Press Inc., New York

British Library Cataloguing in Publication Data
Data available

Library of Congress Cataloging in Publication Data
Data available

Typeset by Newgen Imaging Systems (P) Ltd., Chennai, India
Printed in Italy
on acid-free paper by
L.E.G.O. S.p.A – Lavis TN

ISBN   978–0–19–923028–0

10 9 8 7 6 5 4 3 2 1

Whilst every effort has been made to ensure that the contents of this book are as
complete, accurate and-up-to-date as possible at the date of writing. Oxford
University Press is not able to give any guarantee or assurance that such is the case.
Readers are urged to take appropriately qualified medical advice in all cases. The
information in this book is intended to be useful to the general reader, but should
not be used as a means of self-diagnosis or for the prescription of medication.

O P M L
OXFORD PAIN MANAGEMENT LIBRARY

Chronic Pain

Oxford University Press makes no representation, express or implied, that the drug dosages in this book are correct. Readers must therefore always check the product information and clinical procedures with the most up-to-date published product information and data sheets provided by the manufacturers and the most recent codes of conduct and safety regulations. The authors and the publishers do not accept responsibility or legal liability for any errors in the text or for the misuse or misapplication of material in this work.

▶ Except where otherwise stated, drug doses and recommendations are for the non-pregnant adult who is not breast-feeding.

Contents

Contributors *vii*

1   Chronic non-cancer pain
    Karen H. Simpson   1

2   Paracetamol and Non Steroidal
    Anti-Inflammatory Drugs
    Andrew Dickman and Roger Knaggs   15

3   Tramadol
    Andrew Dickman and Roger Knaggs   25

4   Opioids
    Andrew Dickman and Roger Knaggs   31

5   Antiepileptics
    Andrew Dickman and Roger Knaggs   53

6   Antidepressants
    Andrew Dickman and Roger Knaggs   63

7   Miscellaneous analgesics
    Andrew Dickman and Roger Knaggs   69

8   Interventional techniques for chronic pain
    Brigitta Brandner and M. Nagaratnam   93

9 Non-pharmacological approaches to
   pain management
   Mark I. Johnson and Jan M. Bjordal   119

10 Psychological approaches to chronic pain
   Stephen Morley   131

Index *139*

Contributors

Jan M. Bjordal
Physiotherapist and PhD,
Associate Professor,
Bergen University College,
Bergen, Norway

Brigitta Brandner
Head of Acute Pain Research
Group, University College
London Hospitals,
Mortimer Street,
London, UK

Andrew Dickman
Senior Clinical Pharmacist,
Marie Curie Palliative Care
Institute, Liverpool, and the
Cardiothoracic Centre,
Liverpool, UK

Mark I. Johnson
Professor of Pain and Analgesia
Faculty of Health,
Leeds Metropolitan University,
Leeds, UK

Roger Knaggs
Anaesthetics and Pain
Management Clinical Pharmacist,
Queen's University
Medical Centre,
University Hospital NHS Trust,
Nottingham, UK

Stephen Morley
Professor of Clinical Psychology,
Academic Unit of Psychiatry and
Behavioural Sciences,
University of Leeds,
Leeds, UK

Mayavaty Nagaratnam
Pain and Clinical Research Fellow,
Centre for Anaesthesia,
University College London
Hospital, London, UK

Karen H. Simpson
Consultant in Pain Medicine and
Senior Clinical Lecturer,
Leeds Teaching Hospitals Trust,
Seacroft Hospital, Leeds, UK

Chapter 1

Chronic non-cancer pain

Karen H. Simpson

1.1 Introduction

Pain should be seen in context as a possible symptom of many diseases, so the first role of all health care professionals is to consider pain causation before recommending treatments. Pain may also be regarded as the primary disorder in some chronic conditions such as migraine, post-traumatic nerve damage and chronic low back pain, where pain is the predominating symptom (Niv & Devor, 2004). The International Association for the Study of Pain has defined more than 600 pain syndromes affecting different areas of the body, often with different aetiologies. Some patients have complex pain and their presentation may be both physical and behavioural, thus making assessment difficult. Pain changes, patients develop new problems and behavioural problems may mask systemic diseases. Those with the label 'chronic pain patient' may be disadvantaged if this leads to health care professionals failing to assess and reassess pain causation.

Detailed assessment is therefore an essential prerequisite of successful pain management. A careful history and physical examination is required for each site of pain; this may be supported by the use of validated assessment tools for pain, sleep, function and mood. Not all patients who are referred for pain management have an accurate diagnosis, and some patients need relevant investigations (e.g. blood tests, neurophysiology or imaging). Accurate anatomical diagnosis is particularly important where a nerve blocking or neuromodulation technique is being considered as these are anatomically precise and will offer no analgesia if they miss the affected area. Treatment can then be tailored to the causes of pain. Behavioural issues can also affect the outcome of treatments for chronic pain. Not surprisingly, with such diversity, many chronic pain treatments are not always defined by a well-supported scientific evidence base or provided via integrated care pathways.

1.2 **Definitions**

- **Acute pain** is pain of recent onset and probable limited duration; it usually has an identifiable and causal relationship to injury or disease. Acute pain is transmitted in normal pain pathways as a result of nociceptive stimuli. It acts as a useful warning of tissue damage and its duration is usually relatively brief; it usually resolves with tissue healing and time

- **Chronic pain** is pain that has been present for more than 3 months due to cancer or non-cancer causes. Chronic pain is different to acute pain, because it outlasts the original stimulus and usually serves no useful purpose. It is often accompanied by behavioural and mood changes

- **Disability (World Health Organization 1980)** is any restriction or lack (resulting from an impairment) of ability to perform an activity in the manner or within the range considered normal

- **Handicap (World Health Organization 1980)** is a disadvantage for a given individual, resulting from an impairment or disability that limits or prevents the fulfilment of a role that is normal (depending on age, sex, social and cultural factors) for that individual

- **Nociceptive pain** is caused by actual or potential tissue damage. Classical descriptions of nociception involve cell damage, which releases local mediators that stimulate healthy Aδ and C nerve fibres to transmit pain signals to the spinal cord via the spinothalamic tract to the thalamus and higher centres. Nociceptive mechanisms are much more complex than this; many other pathways are involved in nociceptive processing. The nervous system is not hardwired, but is plastic. It responds to afferent stimulation with neuronal and gene changes that occur rapidly in the periphery, spinal cord and brain. Nociceptive pain can be somatic or visceral. Somatic pains are usually well localized, superficial and often described as acute or sharp in nature. Visceral pains are poorly localized, deep and often described as dull or aching

- **Neuropathic pain** is different to nociceptive pain; it is caused by a primary lesion or dysfunction in nerve fibres, spinal cord or brain. Nerve compression or infiltration leads to altered sensation. Damage to peripheral nerves often leads to pain, e.g. diabetic neuropathy or nerve ischaemia in peripheral vascular disease. When peripheral nerves are involved this is sometimes referred to as deafferentation pain. Damage to autonomic nerves may cause sympathetically maintained pain. Damage to nerves within the central nervous system may cause central pain, e.g. following spinal cord compression, multiple sclerosis or cerebrovascular events. Neuropathic pain can be somatic or visceral. Any of the following are strongly suggestive of neuropathic pain:

- **Allodynia**–pain evoked by a non-painful stimulus; static such as with pressure or dynamic such as with stroking the area
- **Hyperpathia**–an increased reaction to a painful stimulus (often a repetitive stimulus) on the background of an increased pain threshold
- **Hyperalgesia**–a response of exaggerated severity following a painful stimulus.

Neuropathic pain is more common in older people; the population prevalence is about 1%. It comprises about 25% of all referrals to pain clinics in the UK. The diagnosis of neuropathic pain is made by careful clinical history and examination; there are validated scales to assess neuropathic pain, e.g. LANSS (Bennett, 2001). Although there are different mechanisms that can lead to neuropathic pain, its clinical presentation can be variable; this leads to difficulties in assessment and management. Effective pain relief is achieved in less than 50% patients with neuropathic pain (Eisenberg et al., 2005). Neuropathic pain leads to a disproportionate use of health care; its treatment is expensive (Berger et al., 2004). About one-third of patients with chronic neuropathic pain are not receiving any kind of treatment (Finnerup et al., 2005).

- **Breakthrough pain** is a transient exacerbation of pain that occurs either spontaneously or in relation to a specific predictable or unpredictable trigger, experienced by patients who have relatively stable and adequately controlled background pain. Pain that occurs as a result of inadequate background analgesia (i.e. at anytime during the titration phase or towards the end of a dose as analgesic levels decline) is incorrectly referred to as breakthrough pain. There are two types of breakthrough pain:
- **Incident pain** is caused by predictable (e.g. walking, wound dressing and drain removal) or unpredictable (e.g. cough) events. Incident pains can be acute, severe and disabling, but are often short-lived. They commonly do not respond well to oral analgesics. Increasing the dose of background drugs causes sedation when the incident pain is not present. Nerve blocking techniques can be particularly useful in the management of difficult incident pain
- **Spontaneous pain** is unexpected pain with no apparent cause.

3

1.3 **Epidemiology and impact of chronic pain**

Persistent pain is a major problem for patients and poses a massive socio-economic burden for health services and the worldwide community. In Western Europe, chronic pain prevalence is 1 in 5; 70 million adults suffer persistent pain and one-third of households are affected by pain. A European telephone survey of over 46,000 householders showed that 11–30% people had significant chronic pain with profound effects on quality of life for patients and their families (Breivik *et al.*, 2006):

Pain problems persist for many years.

- Young workers are commonly affected
- One-third of patients describe pain as so bad that they could not tolerate any more pain
- 50% feel tired all the time, helpless, older than they really are and could not remember what it feels like not to be in pain
- One-fifth feel that pain is sometimes so bad that they want to die
- One-third reported pain affecting employment
- One-fourth reported losing a job due to pain
- One-fourth were depressed because of pain.

A more detailed assessment was made of subgroups from several countries in this survey. The UK subset (about 300 people) had an average age of 49 years, 70% had pain at least daily; quality of life, mood and capacity to work were all adversely affected by pain. This work supported findings from an earlier UK postal survey of over 5000 adult patients from 29 general practices in Scotland; 50% patients self-reported chronic pain (Elliott *et al.*, 1999). Back pain and arthritis accounted for one-third of all complaints. Logistic-regression modelling identified age, sex, housing tenure and employment status as significant predictors of chronic pain in the community. Pain often persists as shown in a follow-up study of more than 2000 of these patients, 79% of those with pain at initial assessment still had pain 4 years later (Elliott *et al.*, 2000). Therefore it is clear that chronic pain is common, it affects the working population, it often lasts for many years and it impacts on most aspects of function. Unrelieved chronic pain causes interference with daily activities, loss of sleep and increased sickness absence from education or paid employment.

Many studies highlight back pain as a particular problem and this is a good model for considering general issues about the impact of chronic pain.

1–2.5% of the gross national product of many western countries is used to treat musculoskeletal problems.

- Back pain is one of the top 10 most expensive problems
- Back pain is the number one cause of long-term sickness amongst manual workers
- Five million adults consult a doctor about back pain every year
- One-third people aged 16–24 years old report 1–6 days of back pain during a 1-year period
- The direct UK health care cost of back pain in 1998 was £1.6 billion and the cost of informal care and lost production was £10.7 billion
- In 1997/98, 180 million working days were lost due to back pain in the UK
- In Europe, persistent back pain leads to about 500 million lost working days per year and costs in the region of 34 billion Euros
- In 2000, £31 million as spent in Wales on analgesics including £17 million non-steroidal anti-inflammatory drugs
- Failed back surgery syndrome (FBSS) is chronic back or leg pain that persists after technically anatomically successful spinal surgery. FBSS affects three million patients in Europe and occurs in about 40% patients after lumbar spinal surgery (North et al., 2005).

Therefore, persistent back pain is a huge burden and finding effective treatments has important clinical, social, economic and political implications. It is important to address the physical and psychosocial aspects of any chronic pain. In the mid-1980s, work by Waddell, an orthopaedic surgeon, and Main, a clinical psychologist, revealed that the disability associated with chronic non-specific low back pain is only partly explicable in terms of physical factors found on examination (Main & Waddell, 1998). They discovered that psychological factors are almost as significant as contributors to the level of disability. They observed a range of psychological factors that have been shown to play a major part in the development of disability. Negative thoughts, attitudes and emotions (emotional distress) are important factors in the transition from acute to chronic pain states. Chronic pain may lead to depression, anxiety, anger and other psychological problems. It is recognized that psychological factors have a marked influence on pain and disability; these effects may be greater than biomedical factors. Important psychological factors promoting the process of conversion from acute to chronic pain and disability include beliefs about, and attitudes towards, pain, coping strategies, catastrophization and emotional distress. There is often prolonged disability and sometimes problem drug use in those with chronic pain. Clinicians may unwittingly reinforce negative psychological factors, including fear and false beliefs about pain and its cause. Sometimes, the patient's family is involved in the multifaceted pain picture. The activities and attitudes of the family are other important factors, especially those of the spouse or main carer. He or she may reinforce negative thinking and emotion and increase disability by encouraging dependency, albeit unconsciously. Addressing these issues is integral to multidisciplinary pain management.

1.4 Risk factors for chronic pain

- Older age group
- Females
- Poor education
- Unemployment
- Poor general health
- Social disadvantage
- Increased psychological distress.

1.5 Aetiology of chronic pain

This section lists some common general causes of chronic pain and gives some examples of pain types in each category. There are comments on selected topics; these are not intended to be exhaustive, but to provide some insight into relevant issues within each category. More detailed expositions of each type of pain are available in standard texts.

- **Musculoskeletal pain**, e.g. cervical spondylosis, degenerative low back pain, FBSS, osteoarthritis, inflammatory arthritis, polymylagia and myofascial pain syndromes. The most common causes of persistent pain are musculoskeletal; a World Health Organization (WHO) and European Bone and Joint Strategy Project showed:
  - Musculoskeletal pain is the most common reason for primary care consultations leading to 30% of all repeat consultations
  - 60% people on long-term sick leave give musculoskeletal problems as the cause
  - 40% of those aged over 70 years have osteoarthritis of the knees
  - 8–10 million people in the UK have arthritis (12,000 children, 1 million adults under 45 years, 70% of 70 year olds)
  - 80% people report low back pain at some time
  - Musculoskeletal pain sufferers are the second largest group on incapacity benefits.
- **Post-traumatic pain**, e.g. brachial and lumbar plexus injury, vertebral crush fractures and amputation pain
  - Brachial plexus avulsion is a common injury in young men after motor bike accidents. It produces severe neuropathic pain and disability. Although functional improvement can often be achieved by nerve grafts, tendon transfers and reconstructive surgery, pain often persists

- Vertebral crush fractures are a common cause of pain and disability in elderly women and can occur after minimal trauma in those with osteoporosis. Although attention to bone metabolism and appropriate early prophylaxis is important, prevention of falls is a key issue. This influences treatment choices, e.g. avoidance of sedatives and drugs, that cause postural hypotension
- Three separate phenomena can occur after amputation of a body part: phantom sensation, stump pain and phantom pain
- Risk factors for the development of phantom limb pain include persistent stump pain, bilateral and lower limb amputations and pre-amputation pain
- Phantom limb pain is a common and difficult condition to treat. There is insufficient evidence to support the routine use of pre-operative epidural anaesthesia as a technique to prevent phantom limb pain. Surgical revision for stump pain is only indicated when localized pathology is identified.

- **Post-surgical pain**, e.g. after breast surgery, vasectomy, hernia repair, coronary artery bypass, thoracotomy and amputation
  - Persistent pain after surgery is common; it occurs in 10–50% of cases
  - Persistent post-surgical pain is a major clinical problem in about 2–10% of these patients
  - Iatrogenic neuropathic pain is common, so surgical techniques that avoid nerve damage should be used whenever possible.
  - The intensity of acute post-operative pain correlates with the risk of developing persistent pain after surgery.

- **Central pain**, e.g. multiple sclerosis, spinal cord damage, syringomyelia and central post-stroke pain (CPSP)
  - CPSP is a neuropathic pain syndrome characterized by constant or intermittent pain in a body part occurring after stroke and associated with sensory abnormalities in the painful body part
  - CPSP is often under-diagnosed
  - It occurs in 8–10% patients
  - Evoked dysaesthesia and allodynia are common.

- **Peripheral nerve pain**, e.g. peripheral neuropathy and complex regional pain syndrome (CRPS)
  - CRPS is a painful syndrome occurring after an initiating noxious stimulus
  - The provoking event may be a minor injury
  - CRPS I occurs without a definable nerve lesion and CRPS II occurs where there is a definable nerve lesion
  - CRPS affects the limbs but may occur in or spread to other parts of the body

- It includes regional pain, sensory changes (e.g. allodynia), abnormalities of temperature and sudomotor activity, oedema and abnormal skin colour
- Standardized, consensus-based diagnostic criteria for CRPS are important for accurate diagnosis.
- **Facial pain**, e.g. trigeminal neuralgia, temporo-mandibular joint pain and atypical facial pain
  - Trigeminal neuralgia is a rare but characteristic pain syndrome; many cases are associated with vascular compression of the trigeminal nerve
  - A minority of cases are due to multiple sclerosis or nerve compression by tumour
  - Most patients respond well to drugs; carbamazepine is usually the first line treatment
  - Ablative surgical treatments may be associated with corneal/facial sensory loss; severe complications or death are rare but there is a high rate of pain recurrence
  - Microvascular decompression has some risks (severe complications or death) but a lower relapse rate.
- **Headaches**, e.g. tension headache, migraine, cluster headaches and post-traumatic headaches
  - Neuroimaging of headache patients has improved the understanding of the pathophysiology of primary headaches
  - Activation in migraine (brainstem) and in several trigeminal-autonomic headaches (hypothalamic grey) is involved in pain processing
  - No structural changes are seen in migraine and medication overuse headache
  - Patients with chronic tension-type headache show a decrease in grey matter in regions known to be involved in pain processing
  - Most primary headache syndromes are predominantly driven from the brain and need therapies that act centrally and peripherally.
- **Infection**, e.g. HIV-related pains and post-herpetic neuralgia (PHN)
  - Herpes zoster results from re-activation of latent varicella-zoster virus within the sensory ganglia
  - The incidence and severity of herpes zoster increase with advancing age; more than 50% of those who get herpes zoster are older than 60 years
  - The most frequent debilitating complication is PHN; this persistent and often disabling neuropathic pain develops after the dermatomal rash has healed
  - There are many limitations of current therapies for herpes zoster

- A possible way forward is prevention by the use of a live attenuated vaccine; it would be important to target the most vulnerable groups.
- **Vascular pain**, e.g. mesenteric ischaemia, refractory angina, peripheral vascular disease and Raynauds
  - Spinal cord stimulation (SCS) has been used as a treatment for ischaemic conditions
  - Pain relief and limb salvage after SCS in patients with critical non-reconstructable limb ischaemia are significantly higher after 12 months; SCS does not improve ulcer healing
  - There is evidence to favour SCS over standard conservative treatment to improve limb salvage in this group, but the potential benefits of SCS must be weighed against the possible complications and costs.
- **Visceral pain**, e.g. sickle cell pain, pancreatitis, interstitial cystitis and endometriosis
  - Pain is the major presenting symptom of chronic pancreatitis; it is the most important factor affecting quality of life
  - The cause of pain in chronic pancreatitis is multi-factorial; central sensitization and hyperalgesia are important issues
  - Strict abstinence from alcohol is the first step in management
  - Treatable complications, such as pseudocysts, must be dealt with
  - Most patients with chronic pancreatitis require analgesics; care must be taken as problem drug use may occur
  - Meta-analysis shows no significant benefit from pancreatic enzyme supplements for pain.
- **Life-limiting conditions**, e.g. cancer, vascular problems and cerebrovascular problems
  - Pain is one of the most feared symptoms of cancer and other life-limiting diseases
  - Approximately 30–40% of patients with cancer on active therapy report pain; this rises to 70–90% of patients with advanced disease. About 76% of patients with chronic lung disease report pain during the final year of life, with more than half rating pain as 'very distressing'
  - Many studies show that patients with cancer-related pain often have inadequate pain management in hospital
  - 32% of patients with end-stage heart failure and 65% of stroke patients experience pain that is difficult to manage in their last year of life.

1.6 **Pain in children**

Some studies in neonates have suggested that early pain experiences can have an effect on pain perception and painful conditions in adult life. Less is known about the prevalence of pain in children than in adults. One study revealed that of 6000 children at home, 54% had experienced pain within the previous 3 months, and one-fourth of those had had repeated or chronic pain. Pain was most common in the limbs, head and abdomen, and 50% of children had more than one type of pain. Girls over 12 years of age recorded more chronic pain and multiple pains than boys or younger girls. Services for children with chronic pain are poorly established in most countries.

1.7 **Pain in the elderly**

Pain occurs in 45–85% of elderly people; much of it is under treated. Nociception appears not to change with age or with the development of dementia, although a person's perception of pain and willingness to report it may change. Many older people choose not to report their pain for a number of reasons; often they are afraid that they will be hospitalized or subjected to invasive procedures if they report pain. Another important barrier to successful pain management is the fact that older people are often misinformed about the aging process, analgesics, pain management and opioid addiction. Pain leads to poor quality of life, sleep disturbances, cognitive impairment, malnutrition, decreased socialization and depression. The management of pain in elderly patients is often complicated by the changing physiology that occurs with aging. Older people are also more likely to be living with multiple chronic diseases (Robinson, 2007). The need for poly-pharmacy increases the risk drug interactions. As a patient's number of medications increases, so does the risk of adverse reactions; therefore, care is required when adding any new medication to the drug regimen. Achieving adequate pain management for the older patient is therefore complicated by co-morbid diseases, increased risk of adverse drug reactions, and physician factors such as inadequate training in pain medicine and a reluctance to prescribe opioid medications.

1.8 **Pain in vulnerable groups**

Certain groups are disadvantaged in terms of pain assessment and management, often because of failures in communication and the beliefs of the health care professionals. Patients with learning difficulties, those with special needs, nursing home residents, prisoners, refugees, victims of abuse or torture and survivors of wars are all at risk.

These groups have special requirements that may be difficult to manage; however, it is important to be sensitive to their needs and to strive to improve services for them. Often simple measures such as the choice of appropriate assessment tools (e.g. pain scales in multiple languages (British Pain Society, 2007) faces pictorial scales), the provision of interpreters and allowing adequate time for assessment and explanation go a long way to improving their care. It is not usually the lack of high technology strategies, but poor attention to basic principles that leads to them being denied access to good care.

1.9 **Effective pain management**

Most pain management for cancer and non-cancer chronic pain happens in primary care. Therefore, community-based services need adequate education and support from specialist pain services to deal with this common, but difficult, clinical problem. All pain management teams should support community care to patients with a wide range of different chronic pain conditions. It is important that primary care and secondary care are integrated if persistent pain is to be managed well. Acceptance of agreed and evidence-based local care pathways for common chronic pain problems would go a long way to helping those with persistent pain.

Basic chronic pain management services are needed within all secondary care services. There should be selective provision of specialist pain management services on a regional basis and for cancer centres; specialist pain management and palliative care services provide clinically effective care at a low cost. Efficient and effective pain management requires established links between secondary care medical specialties, e.g. surgery, medicine, rheumatology, gastroenterology, neurology, elderly medicine, rehabilitation medicine, occupational health, oncology, palliative medicine, psychiatry, addiction medicine and paediatrics.

Pain management uses a multidisciplinary team approach that matches therapy to the individual patient. Good pain management needs interdisciplinary co-operation among health care professionals, e.g. doctors, specialist nurses, dieticians, clinical psychologists, physiotherapists, pharmacists, social workers and occupational therapists. Patients with chronic pain have complex bio-psychosocial problems that cannot be addressed with unimodal therapy; pain services should provide a range of treatments:

- Pharmacological therapies should be seen as a part of an integrated plan to improve physical and social functions and support a rehabilitative approach. The emphasis must be on medication management to underpin functional restoration. Pharmacists and specialist pain nurses have a vital role in medication management and follow up

- Rehabilitation should involve setting clear goals, with plans for steady progress towards them. There are many systematic reviews on the use of analgesic drugs and techniques and it is essential to balance the benefits and burdens of such treatments carefully because chronic pain management is often long-term

- Effective relief of pain is usually obtained with oral or sometimes transdermal drugs; therefore, it is important to use the most effective and safest route available. The use of immediate release opioids or injectable analgesics in chronic pain must be discouraged, as this approach often creates more problems than it solves

- Nerve blocks or neuromodulation should form part of a strategy aimed at pain management, functional restoration and rehabilitation. There is no point using physical techniques alone to manage pain that has significant non-physical elements. A careful assessment at the outset will avoid subjecting a patient to an invasive procedure with little chance of benefit. Decision-making is dependent on good communication both within a team and between teams when a nerve block or neuromodulation technique is being considered. Interventions may need to be performed urgently, but are rarely needed as an emergency. It is important that patients are given time to think about the options and to ask questions; written information can be very helpful

- Various physical interventions can be used to manage chronic pain. Some therapies involve stimulation of the nervous system, while others rely on mobilizations and exercise, e.g. transcutaneous electrical nerve stimulation (TENS) or acupuncture. Most have the advantage of avoiding drug side effects and promoting patients' self-efficacy. Physiotherapists, occupational therapists, osteopaths, chiropractors, acupuncturists and specialist nurses have important roles in delivering many of these therapies

- An important part of this is teaching patients with pain about regular, paced exercise and reducing maladaptive behaviours, e.g. fear avoidance. All health care professionals involved in managing persistent pain should address behaviours and coping styles that increase disability and dependence. Some patients benefit from individual or group work with a clinical psychologist who may use a variety of strategies; cognitive behavioural therapy is commonly used (Morley & Keefe, 2007)

- Pain services provide treatments for pain, but as importantly have an educational role for patients and their carers. It is important that patients understand the difference between acute and chronic pain and have any misconceptions about the meaning of pain explained. Much of the work of chronic pain services is to reduce disability and improve function by helping patients overcome their fears about what pain means. As well as explaining pain mechanisms and treatment strategies to patients, written information should be available explaining the treatments available in the pain management unit in a way that is readily understandable. This must cater for all patients, including those with special requirements. Patients must be able to make an informed decision about the pain management treatments that they choose.

1.10 **Summary**

Integrated and shared care is important in managing all chronic conditions and pain is no exception. The following principles are important:

- Assess and treat each cause of pain
- Primary management involves establishing and reversing the cause of the pain where possible or modifying the disease process if the cause cannot be removed
- Remove or reduce exacerbating factors, e.g. paced activity
- Explore the meaning of the pain for the patient, e.g. worsening symptoms may be equated with the progression of disease and fear of dependency and disability
- Modify the social/physical environment where relevant, e.g. appropriate mattresses, orthotics, chairs, wheelchairs, stair lifts and bathing facilities. Working to maintain or introduce hobbies and interests in addition to enhancing the social environment may contribute to improving coping styles and enhancing quality of life
- Treat mood disorders, e.g. depression and/or anxiety using drug or non-drug measures as appropriate
- Use regular oral analgesics and co-analgesics if appropriate
- Nerve blocks or neuromodulation techniques may be needed in a small number of patients
- Physical therapies provide advantages such as safety and self-efficacy
- Psychological strategies are an important aspect of chronic pain management
- The needs of patients and families with chronic pain must be defined
- Multidisciplinary teams should integrate generalist and specialist expertise
- Care must be coordinated across organizational boundaries
- Unnecessary visits and admissions to hospital should be avoided
- Care should occur in the most appropriate setting for the patient and the procedure
- Care pathways for common chronic pain conditions need to be developed and implemented (Bandolier Forum, 2003; Tsai *et al.*, 2005).

Key references

Bandolier Forum (July 2003). *On Care Pathways*. Available from www.ebandolier.com.

Bennett M (2001). The LANSS Pain Scale: the Leeds assessment of neuropathic symptoms and signs. *Pain* **92**: 147–57.

Berger A, Dukes EM, Oster G (2004). Clinical characteristics and economic costs of patients with painful neuropathic disorders. *J. Pain* **5**: 143–9.

Breivik H, Collett B, Ventafridda V, *et al.* (2006). Survey of chronic pain in Europe: prevalence, impact on daily life, and treatment. *Eur. J. Pain* **10**: 287–333.

Eisenberg E, McNicol ED, Carr DB (2005). Efficacy and safety of opioid agonists in the treatment of neuropathic pain of non-malignant origin: systematic review and meta-analysis of randomized controlled trials. *JAMA* **293**: 3043–52.

Elliott AM, Smith BH, Penny KI, *et al.* (1999). The epidemiology of chronic pain in the community. *Lancet* **354**: 1248–52.

Elliott AM, Smith BH, Smith WC, Chambers WA (2000). Changes in chronic pain severity over time: the Chronic Pain Grade as a valid measure. *Pain* **88**: 303–8.

Finnerup NB, Otto M, McQuay HJ, *et al.* (2005). Algorithm for neuropathic pain treatment: an evidence based proposal. *Pain* **118**: 289–305.

Main CJ, Waddell G (1998). Behavioural responses to examination. A reappraisal of the interpretation of "non-organic signs". *Spine* **23**: 2367–71.

Morley S, Keefe FJ (2007). Getting a handle on process and change in CBT for chronic pain. *Pain* **127**: 197–8.

Niv D, Devor M (2004). Chronic pain as a disease in its own right. *Pain Pract.* **4**: 179–81.

North RB, Kidd DH, Farrokhi F, Piantadosi SA (2005). Spinal cord stimulation versus repeated lumbosacral spine surgery for chronic pain: a randomized, controlled trial. *Neurosurgery* **56**: 98–106; discussion 106–7.

Robinson CL (2007). Relieving pain in the elderly. *Health Prog.* **88**: 48–53.

The British Pain Society (2007). *Pain Scales in Multiple Languages*. Available from http://www.britishpainsociety.org/pub_pain_scales.htm (accessed 1 September 2007).

Tsai AC, Morton SC, Mangione CM, Keeler EB (2005). A meta-analysis of interventions to improve care for chronic illness. *Am. J. Manag. Care* **11**: 478–88.

Chapter 2

Paracetamol and Non Steroidal Anti-Inflammatory Drugs

Andrew Dickman and Roger Knaggs

Key points

- Paracetamol is a useful analgesic for mild to moderate pain
- Its widespread availability should not infer ineffectiveness
- Paracetamol can be opioid sparing and should be considered the simple analgesic of choice
- Each patient should be carefully assessed before a NSAID or COX-2 inhibitor is prescribed
- COX-2 inhibitors must not be used in patients with established ischaemic heart disease, peripheral vascular disease and/or cerebrovascular disease.

Simple analgesics, e.g. paracetamol (acetaminophen) and non-steroidal anti-inflammatory drugs (NSAIDs), are often considered as step 1 on the World Health Organization analgesic ladder. Although this tool was primarily developed for cancer pain, its general principles can be adapted to non-cancer pains. Simple analgesics have no activity at opioid receptors and therefore do not induce tolerance and dependence that sometimes occurs with opioids. However, when used in combination with opioids there is synergistic analgesia, so they may be opioid sparing.

2.1 Paracetamol

Paracetamol (acetaminophen) is a derivative of aniline, a constituent of coal tar. It is effective with a good safety profile. Earlier attempts to use related compounds, e.g. phenacetin, were not successful due to the methaemoglobin toxicity. Paracetamol is useful for mild to moderate pain. It is antipyretic. It is not an anti-inflammatory.

2.1.1 Pharmacology

Although the mechanism of action remains uncertain, there are data to suggest a central nervous system site of action. Aniline derivatives have strong antipyretic effects mediated in the thermoregulatory centre in the hypothalamus. Paracetamol is a small, lipophilic molecule that crosses the human blood–brain barrier (Bannworth *et al.*, 1992). Paracetamol may inhibit cyclooxygenases (COX-1 and COX-2) within the central nervous system, but this has been difficult to demonstrate. A COX-3 variant and potential target for paracetamol has been postulated (Chandrasekharan *et al.*, 2002).

There has been interest in the effect of paracetamol in modulating the serotoninergic (5-HT) neurotransmitter system (Pelissier *et al.*, 1996). Clinical experience suggests that its combination with an opioid may reduce the opioid dose, indicating potentiation or modulation of endogenous opioid systems.

Paracetamol is quickly absorbed from the gastrointestinal (GI) tract after oral administration; it has a bioavailability of around 60%. Analgesic plasma concentrations are attained in 15–30 minutes; peak concentrations are reached within 1 hour if gastric emptying is normal. The plasma elimination half-life is approximately 3 hours. Analgesia lasts up to 6 hours. After rectal administration, its bioavailability is considerably lower and absorption is often delayed and erratic.

2.1.2 **Contraindications and precautions**

- Hepatic and renal impairment
- Alcohol dependence
- Use of paracetamol during pregnancy or breastfeeding is not known to be harmful.

2.1.3 **Adverse effects**

Paracetamol is generally well-tolerated, although there have been rare reports of rashes, blood dyscrasias and liver damage.

Important

Paracetamol toxicity

Both acute and chronic toxicity may develop following paracetamol administration.

Acute toxicity

A minor route of paracetamol metabolism is through a cytochrome P450 mediated reaction that forms a reactive intermediate, N-acteyl-p-benzoquinimine (NAPQI). Usually, NAPQI can be deactivated by conjugation with glutathione in the liver. However, following ingestion of a large amount of paracetamol the hepatic stores of glutathione become depleted so more NAPQI is available to cause hepatic damage by arylating and oxidizing hepatocellular proteins, leading to inhibition of enzyme activity and cellular death. Toxicity may occur following ingestion of approximately twice the normal daily dose (i.e. 14–16 paracetamol 500 mg tablets in an adult).

(Contd.)

A small number of people may be at high risk of acute paracetamol toxicity; this includes patients who are malnourished for any reason (e.g. anorexia, AIDS and cancer), alcoholics, or those taking hepatic enzyme inducing drugs (e.g. many of the older antiepileptics).

Chronic toxicity

Paracetamol has tenuously been linked to causing renal damage and hypertension, particularly in women, with long-term use. The precise mechanism of chronic renal toxicity remains unclear, although may involve renal cell death and deterioration of tubular function. Further evidence is needed before widespread changes to practice need to occur.

2.1.4 **Drug interactions**

Cases of enhancement of warfarin action with chronic paracetamol therapy have been reported.

2.1.5 **Administration**

Paracetamol is most commonly administered orally and is available as tablets, capsules and as oral suspension. Rectal administration is an alternative if the oral route is unavailable although absorption is erratic. The usual adult dose is 500–1000 mg every 4–6 hours, with a maximum of 4000 mg daily. Daily doses above 4000 mg are likely to result in toxicity. An injectable preparation is available that is mainly used in acute pain and is not likely to have a major role in chronic pain.

There are many over the counter preparations and several prescription products that contain paracetamol in addition to other drugs. Compound preparations (e.g. co-codamol and co-dydramol) containing varying amounts of paracetamol and a weak opioid are not recommended for routine prescribing; their opioid content is generally too low to be analgesic but sufficient to cause side effects. The exception to this is Tramacet® that has been shown to be an effective combination of paracetamol and the opioid tramadol. Co-methiamol (methionine 100 mg, paracetamol 500 mg) is also available; methionine binds to NAPQI and may prevent paracetamol toxicity in the event of overdose.

2.2 **Non-steroidal anti-inflammatory drugs**

NSAIDs are a heterogeneous group and are the commonest analgesics prescribed worldwide. They are generally well-tolerated and provide effective relief for mild to moderate pain (McNicol *et al.*, 2005; Zhang *et al.*, 2005); they all have antipyretic and anti-inflammatory actions.

2.2.1 **Pharmacology**

The primary mechanism of action of all the NSAIDs is the inhibition of prostaglandin biosynthesis; prostaglandins are one of the major components of the 'inflammatory soup' that sensitizes peripheral nociceptors. Prostaglandins have diverse homeostatic functions (Figure 2.1) in addition to a role in inflammation. Prostaglandins PGE_2 and PGI_2 are both involved in inflammatory pain. Prostaglandins sensitize peripheral $A\delta$ and C nerve fibres to mechanical stimulation and other inflammatory mediators, including histamine and bradykinin. Inhibition of PGI_2 (prostacyclin) synthesis is implicated as the major cause of the renal and cardiovascular adverse effects of the NSAIDs.

Prostaglandins are synthesized as a result of the enzymatic breakdown of arachidonic acid, a constituent of mammalian cell membranes that is catalysed by COX; NSAIDs inhibit this enzyme. Aspirin irreversibly binds to the enzyme and all other non-salicylate NSAIDs are reversible COX inhibitors (Smith, 1992). Towards the end of the 20th Century at least two isoforms of this enzyme, COX-1 and COX-2, were identified. It was believed that COX-1 was constitutive having a regulatory role (e.g. gastric homeostasis) and COX-2 was inducible at sites of inflammation. The anti-inflammatory, antipyretic and analgesic actions of NSAIDs were associated with inhibition of COX-2 and the adverse effects were associated with inhibition of COX-1.

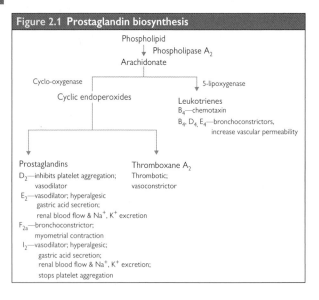

Figure 2.1 Prostaglandin biosynthesis

Phospholipid
$\downarrow$ Phospholipase A_2
Arachidonate

Cyclo-oxygenase   5-lipoxygenase

Cyclic endoperoxides   Leukotrienes
B_4—chemotaxin
B_4, D_4, E_4—bronchoconstrictors, increase vascular permeability

Prostaglandins   Thromboxane A_2
D_2—inhibits platelet aggregation;   Thrombotic;
    vasodilator   vasoconstrictor
E_2—vasodilator; hyperalgesic
    gastric acid secretion;
    renal blood flow & Na^+, K^+ excretion
F_{2a}—bronchoconstrictor;
    myometrial contraction
I_2—vasodilator; hyperalgesic;
    gastric acid secretion;
    renal blood flow & Na^+, K^+ excretion;
    stops platelet aggregation

Unfortunately, this was not the complete picture and even now the action of the NSAIDs is still not completely understood. COX-2 has a constitutive role within the kidney (salt and water balance), vascular endothelium (vasodilation and inhibition of platelet aggregation) and GI tract (mucosal protection), which explains the adverse effects that the COX-2 inhibitors display. The discovery of COX-3 complicates the situation further.

The majority of older NSAIDs (e.g. diclofenac and naproxen) inhibit both COX-1 and COX-2 to a greater or lesser extent. Newer NSAIDs (e.g. meloxicam and etodolac) are more selective for the COX-2 isoform. This selectivity has been developed further with COX-2 selective drugs (e.g. celecoxib, etoricoxib).

All NSAIDs are almost completely absorbed after oral dosing; however, the rate of absorption is altered by changes in GI blood flow or motility and/or if the drug is taken with food. Some NSAIDs have been formulated with an enteric coat to reduce the direct irritant effect on the GI mucosa but this may also lower the rate of absorption. Most NSAIDs are weak organic acids, so absorption begins from the stomach; however due to its large surface area, the small intestine is the main site of absorption.

Following absorption, there is significant binding to plasma proteins, including albumin (>95% in most cases). Reduction in the amount of plasma albumin will result in more unbound drug in the systemic circulation with potential additional adverse effects. NSAIDs are predominately metabolized by the hepatic cytochrome P450 enzyme system before being excreted in the urine. Several NSAIDs undergo significant enterohepatic recycling that prolongs the elimination half-life.

There are marked differences in plasma elimination half-life for individual NSAIDs and this may be important in explaining differences in clinical effect. NSAIDs with a long half-life, e.g. piroxicam ($t_{1/2}$ 5–22 hours), do not achieve maximum plasma concentrations quickly, so it takes a long time to reach therapeutic effect. Although a long half-life with longer dosing intervals may improve patient concordance, it does not benefit patients at risk of NSAID-induced toxicity (e.g. the elderly).

2.2.2 Contraindications and precautions

Non-selective NSAIDs must not be used in patients with:

- active, or a history of, GI ulcers, bleeding or perforation (two or more distinct episodes of proven ulceration or bleeding)
- a history of GI bleeding or perforation, relating to previous NSAID therapy
- inflammatory bowel disease

- previous hypersensitivity reactions (e.g. asthma, angioedema, urticaria or acute rhinitis) to ibuprofen, aspirin or other NSAIDs
- severe hepatic, renal or heart failure
- porphyria (check individual drugs)
- pregnancy (especially third trimester).

COX-2 selective inhibitors must not be used in patients with:
- active peptic ulceration or GI bleeding
- established ischaemic heart disease, peripheral arterial disease and/or cerebrovascular disease
- if a patient has experienced asthma, acute rhinitis, nasal polyps, angioneurotic oedema, urticaria or other allergic-type reactions after taking acetylsalicylic acid or NSAIDs or COX-2 selective inhibitors
- severe hepatic, renal or heart failure
- inflammatory bowel disease
- porphyria (check individual drugs)
- pregnancy and breastfeeding.

The following precautions apply to non-selective NSAID use:
- Patients with uncontrolled hypertension, congestive heart failure, established ischaemic heart disease, peripheral arterial disease and/or cerebrovascular disease need careful consideration due to the increased risk of thrombotic events
- Similar consideration should be made before initiating longer-term treatment of patients with risk factors for cardiovascular events (e.g. hypertension, hyperlipidaemia, diabetes mellitus and smoking)
- Caution should be exercised in patients with a history of cardiac failure, left ventricular dysfunction or hypertension. Deterioration may occur due to fluid retention
- Patients taking long-term therapy need regular monitoring of renal and liver functions
- Caution in patients with impaired cardiac or renal function, those being treated with diuretics and those recovering from major surgery
- Abnormal liver functions tests can occur; discontinue NSAID if this persists
- Patients with haematological disorders should be closely monitored
- Skin reactions may occur and are generally evident within the first month of treatment; these can be fatal
- Breastfeeding—diclofenac and ibuprofen are unlikely to be harmful.

The following precautions apply to COX-2 selective inhibitors:

- Caution in the elderly, patients using any other NSAID or aspirin concomitantly, or patients with a prior history of GI disease (including previous peptic ulcer). These patients are most at risk of developing GI complications
- The cardiovascular risks may increase with dose and duration of exposure; use the shortest duration and the lowest effective daily dose possible
- Caution in patients with risk factors for cardiovascular events (e.g. hypertension, hyperlipidaemia, diabetes mellitus and smoking)
- Caution in patients with a history of cardiac failure, left ventricular dysfunction or hypertension. Deterioration may occur due to fluid retention
- Caution in patients with impaired cardiac or renal function. Monitoring of renal function should be considered
- Abnormal liver functions tests can occur; discontinue if this persists
- Skin reactions that are generally evident within the first month of treatment may occur; these can be fatal.

2.2.3 **Adverse effects**

Inhibition of COX-1 and COX-2 mediated homeostatic synthesis of prostaglandins results in a wide range of adverse effects:

- GI tract (risk factors for NSAID-induced GI effects; see Table 2.1)
    - dyspepsia (frequently leads to discontinuation)
    - abdominal pain
    - nausea and vomiting
    - diarrhoea
    - peptic ulcer disease
    - GI bleeding
    - bowel obstruction.
- Renal
    - water and electrolyte retention (sequelae are hypertension and worsening congestive heart failure)
    - reversible acute renal failure.
- Cardiovascular system (Table 2.2)
    - ischaemic heart disease and stroke
    - increased risk of bleeding.
- Respiratory
    - exacerbation of asthma in sensitive individuals.
- Other
    - skin reactions (rare—Stevens-Johnson syndrome)
    - photosensitivity.

Table 2.1 Risk factors for NSAID-induced gastroduodenal damage
• Choice of NSAID
• Dose and duration of NSAID therapy
• Age >65 years
• Use of concurrent medications (e.g. low-dose aspirin, warfarin, corticosteroid and selective serotonin re-uptake inhibitors)
• Previous history of peptic ulcer disease

Table 2.2 Cardiovascular safety information for NSAIDs (February 2008)
• Non-selective NSAIDs and COX-2 selective inhibitors may be associated with a small increased risk of thrombotic events
• For all NSAIDs, thrombotic risk is likely to be greater when used at high doses and for long-term treatment
• The risk may vary between individual drugs
• For non-selective NSAIDs, the absolute risk is currently unknown; for COX-2 selective inhibitors, evidence suggests about three additional thrombotic events may occur per 1000 patients per year
• Naproxen is associated with a risk lower than COX-2 selective drugs
• Diclofenac has a similar risk as etoricoxib.
• Low dose ibuprofen (<1.2 g daily) is believed not to carry significant risk
• Piroxicam is believed to have an increased risk compared to other non-selective NSAIDs.

2.2.4 **Drug interactions**

Pharmacodynamic interactions with NSAIDs and COX-2 inhibitors include:

- ACE inhibitors—Risk of nephrotoxicity and reduced therapeutic effect
- Anticoagulants and antiplatelet drugs—Increased risk of GI bleed
- Antihypertensives—Loss of blood pressure control
- Low-dose aspirin—Potential reduction in antiplatelet effect
- Ciclosporin—Risk of nephrotoxicity
- Corticosteroids—Increased risk of peptic ulceration and GI bleed
- Pentoxifylline—Increased risk of GI bleed
- Selective serotonin-reuptake inhibitors (SSRIs)—Increased risk of GI bleed.

Pharmacokinetic interactions with NSAIDs and COX-2 inhibitors include:

- Anticoagulants—Enhanced effect due to displacement from plasma proteins
- Ciclosporin—Halve dose of *diclofenac*
- Fluconazole—Halve dose of *celecoxib*
- Lithium—Increased risk of toxicity
- Methotrexate—Increased risk of toxicity
- Quinolone antibiotics—Risk of convulsions.

2.2.5 Administration

NSAIDs have been formulated for administration by a variety of routes. The oral route is the most common, and is the preferred route for both acute and chronic administration. See page 87 for topical NSAIDs.

A smaller number of NSAIDs (e.g. diclofenac and ketorolac) have been marketed as injections for parenteral use.

Important

Minimizing NSAID-induced adverse effects

- Consider non-pharmacological measures or other analgesics with fewer side effects (e.g. weak opioid or tramadol)
- The lowest effective dose of NSAID or COX-2 selective inhibitor should be prescribed for the shortest time necessary
- The need for long-term treatment should be reviewed periodically
- Prescribing should be based on the safety of individual NSAIDs or COX-2 selective inhibitors, on individual patient risks (e.g. GI and cardiovascular) and patient preference
- Concomitant aspirin (and possibly other anti-platelet drugs) greatly increases the GI risks of NSAIDs and severely reduces any GI safety advantages of COX-2 selective inhibitors. Aspirin should only be co-prescribed if absolutely necessary
- Consider the use of gastroprotective strategies (misoprostol and proton pump inhibitors have the most evidence)
- Consider checking renal function before and soon after initiating therapy (e.g. after 5 days).

Key references

Bannworth B, Netter P, Lapicque F, *et al.* (1992). Plasma and cerebrospinal concentrations of paracetamol after a single intravenous dose of propacetamol. *Br. J. Clin. Pharmacol.* **24**: 79–81.

Chandrasekharan NV, Dai H, Roos KL, *et al.* (2002). COX-3, a cyclooxygenase-1 variant inhibited by acetaminophen and other analgesic/antipyretic drugs: cloning, structure and expression. *Proc. Natl Acad. Sci. USA* **99**: 13926–31.

McNicol E, Strassels SA, Goudas L, *et al.* (2005). NSAIDS or paracetamol, alone or combined with opioids, for cancer pain. *Cochrane Database Syst. Rev.* **2**: CD005180.

Pelissier T, Alloui A, Caussade F, *et al.* (1996). Paracetamol exerts a spinal antinociceptive effect involving an indirect interaction with 5-hydroxy tryptamine 3 receptors: in vivo and in vitro evidence. *J. Pharmacol. Exp. Ther.* **278**: 8–14.

Smith WL (1992). Prostanoid biosynthesis and mechanisms of action. *Am. J. Physiol.* **263**: F181–96.

Zhang W, Doherty M, Arden N, *et al.* (2005). EULAR evidence based recommendations for the management of hip osteoarthritis: report of a task force of the EULAR standing committee for international clinical studies including therapeutics (ESCISIT). *Ann. Rheum. Dis.* **64**: 669–81.

Chapter 3

Tramadol

Andrew Dickman and Roger Knaggs

Key points

- Tramadol has a complex mechanism of action involving both serotonin/noradrenaline re-uptake inhibition and opioid activity
- An understanding of its pharmacology is essential for successful treatment
- Its opioid effect requires hepatic activation via cytochrome CYP2D6
- Genetic variation and drug interactions can alter both the analgesic and adverse effect profiles.

3.1 Introduction

Tramadol was launched in the UK in 1994 and it is one of the most widely prescribed drugs worldwide. The clinical efficacy of tramadol has been established in numerous studies in chronic pain, e.g. cancer pain and neuropathic pain (Grond et al., 1999; Hollingshead et al., 2006; Arbaiza & Vidal, 2007).

3.2 Pharmacology

Tramadol is a centrally acting analgesic with a unique and complex pharmacology (see Figure 3.1). Analgesia is produced by a synergistic interaction between two distinct pharmacological effects (Ide et al., 2006). Tramadol has a μ-opioid effect. It also activates descending anti-nociceptive pathways in the spinal cord via inhibition of re-uptake of serotonin and noradrenaline and via pre-synaptic release of serotonin. The pharmacology of tramadol may explain its effectiveness in types of pain that are traditionally considered to be poorly opioid responsive, e.g. neuropathic pain.

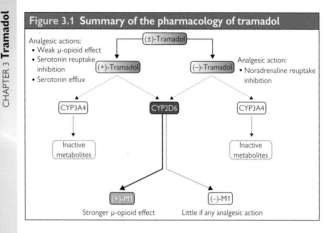

Figure 3.1 Summary of the pharmacology of tramadol

Tramadol is available commercially as a racemate, consisting of enantiomers, (+) tramadol and (−) tramadol that have different pharmacological actions. Opioid and serotonergic actions are associated with (+) tramadol, whereas noradrenaline re-uptake inhibition is associated with (−) tramadol. Racemic (±) tramadol binds to the μ-opioid receptor 6000 times less strongly than morphine, and 10 times less than codeine. The only pharmacologically active metabolite (+) O-desmethyltramadol (or (+) M1) is produced by the polymorphic cytochrome CYP2D6. (+) M1 binds to the μ-opioid receptor with an affinity that is 700 times greater than (±) tramadol. The opioid effect of (±) tramadol is mostly due to (+) M1, as (−) M1 appears devoid of analgesic activity. Additional metabolism of (±) tramadol is catalysed by CYP3A4 to (±) N-desmethyltramadol or (±) M2. Subsequent metabolism of (±) M1 and (±) M2 occurs through processes involving CYP2B6 and CYP3A4 (Grond & Sablotzki, 2004).

Studies suggest that the analgesic effect of (±) tramadol is greater than the sum of its parts; the two enantiomers, together with (+) M1, may act synergistically via spinal modulation and via opioid activity (Raffa et al., 1992; Grond et al., 1995). This synergism is subjected to disruption because the analgesic effect of (±) tramadol is dependent on its metabolism. Genetic variances can encode for several forms of cytochrome CYP2D6 that have varying degrees of activity. Individuals completely lacking CYP2D6 activity are called poor metabolizers who cannot produce (+) M1. Drug interactions can affect the metabolism of (±) tramadol via enzyme inhibition or induction (CYP2D6 cannot be induced). The clinical consequences of genotype and drug interaction depend on the type of pain being treated as the monoaminergic and opioid effects both independently produce analgesia. Genetic variations lead to the possibility of a modified adverse effect profile and reduced analgesic response with tramadol (Stamer *et al.*, 2003).

3.3 Contraindications and precautions

- Avoid in patients who are receiving monoamine oxidase (MAO) inhibitors, or within 2 weeks of their discontinuation
- Tramadol should be used with caution in patients with a history of:
  - head injury
  - raised intracranial pressure
  - epilepsy
  - porphyria.
- Tramadol should only be used if potential benefits outweigh potential risks during pregnancy. It is not teratogenic but very high doses may affect foetal development. Chronic use can cause withdrawal syndrome in newborn
- Breastfeeding is contraindicated if the use of tramadol exceeds more than 3 days.

3.4 Adverse effects

The commonest adverse effect with tramadol is nausea and vomiting, which is most probably due to the serotonergic activity of (+) tramadol rather than its opioid effect. Emesis is more commonly encountered with the immediate release preparation. In patients with chronic pain, the use of the modified release formulation for titration reduces adverse effects and improves tolerability (Tagarro *et al.*, 2005). Tramadol can cause convulsions at therapeutic doses, often when combined with other seizure-threshold lowering drugs (e.g. tricyclic antidepressants). Patients with a history of epilepsy or those susceptible to seizures should only be treated with tramadol if there are compelling reasons (electronic Medicines Compendium, 2007).

3.5 Drug interactions

3.5.1 Pharmacokinetic

The analgesic effect of tramadol may be reduced by co-administration of CYP2D6 inhibitors including (Laugesen *et al.*, 2005):

- paroxetine
- duloxetine

- fluoxetine
- haloperidol
- levomepromazine.

The clinical implications of co-administration of tramadol with these drugs are unknown (except with paroxetine), so clinicians should be alert to the possibility of reduced analgesia and altered adverse effects with tramadol.

Carbamazepine is a CYP3A4 inducer and it reduces the analgesic benefit of tramadol (Grond & Sablotzki, 2004); presumably this occurs through an increase in N-demethylation and subsequent reduction of (±) tramadol and (+) M1.

3.5.2 **Pharmacodynamic**

Combination of tramadol with serotonergic drugs can lead to increased adverse effects, e.g. emesis, or rarely the serotonin syndrome. Such drugs include:

- citalopram
- duloxetine
- fluoxetine
- MAO-inhibitors
- paroxetine
- venlafaxine.

Combination with *tricyclic antidepressants* can increase the risk of seizures in susceptible individuals.

Ondansetron may reduce the analgesic benefit of tramadol through direct antagonism of 5-HT$_3$ receptor mediated analgesia. Nausea and vomiting associated with tramadol have successfully been treated with metoclopramide, with no reduction in analgesia being reported (Pang *et al.*, 2002).

3.6 **Administration**

Tramadol is available as immediate release and modified release oral formulations, as well as a solution for intravenous and intramuscular injections. Although unlicensed, tramadol can be given subcutaneously. The usual maximum daily dose of tramadol is 400 mg. For chronic pain, titrating analgesia requirements with a modified release formulation greatly improves the tolerability of tramadol, e.g. 50 mg twice daily increasing to 100 mg twice daily several days later, with further dose increases as necessary (Tagarro *et al.*, 2005).

Key references

Arbaiza D, Vidal O (2007). Tramadol in the treatment of neuropathic cancer pain. *Clin. Drug Invest.* **27**: 75–83.

Zydol 50 mg capsules [Grünenthal Ltd – Summary of Product Characteristics]. Datapharm Communications Ltd, Surrey. Available from http://emc. medicines.org.uk (accessed on 2 May 2007).

Grond S, Sablotzki A (2004). Clinical pharmacology of tramadol. *Clin. Pharmacokinet.* **43**: 879–923.

Grond S, Meuser T, Zech D, et al. (1995). Analgesic efficacy and safety of tramadol enantiomers in comparison with the racemate: a randomised, double-blind study with gynaecological patients using intravenous patient-controlled analgesia. *Pain* **62**: 313–320.

Grond S, Radbruch L, Meuser T, et al. (1999). High-dose tramadol in comparison to low-dose morphine for cancer pain relief. *J. Pain. Symptom Manage.* **18**: 174–9.

Hollingshead J, Duhmke RM, Cornblath DR (2006). Tramadol for neuropathic pain. *Cochrane Database Syst. Rev.* **19** (3): CD003726.

Ide S, Minami M, Ishihara K, et al. (2006). Mu opioid receptor-dependent and independent components in effects of tramadol. *Neuropharmacology* **51**: 651–8.

Laugesen S, Enggaard TP, Pedersen RS, et al. (2005). Paroxetine, a cytochrome P450 2D6 inhibitor, diminishes the stereoselective O-demethylation and reduces the hypoalgesic effect of tramadol. *Clin. Pharmacol. Ther.* **77**: 312–23.

Pang WW, Wu HS, Lin CH, et al. (2002). Metoclopramide decreases emesis but increases sedation in tramadol patient-controlled analgesia. *Can. J. Anesth.* **49**: 1029–33.

Raffa RB, Friderichs E, Reimann W, Shank RP, et al. (1992). Opioid and nonopioid components independently contribute to the mechanism of action if tramadol, an 'atypical' opioid analgesic. *J. Pharmacol. Exp. Ther.* **260**: 275–85.

Stamer UM, Lehnen K, Hothker F, et al. (2003). Impact of CYP2D6 genotype on postoperative tramadol analgesia. *Pain* **105**: 231–8.

Tagarro I, Herrera J, Barutell C, et al. (2005). Effect of a simple dose-escalation schedule on tramadol tolerability. *Clin. Drug. Invest.* **25**: 23–31.

Chapter 4

Opioids

Andrew Dickman and Roger Knaggs

Key points

- Opioids can be used successfully in the management of chronic non-cancer pain
- A single practitioner should be responsible for prescribing opioids
- Long-term opioid use may be associated with complications such as endocrine and immune dysfunctions.
- The regular use of short-acting opioids for the treatment of chronic non-cancer pain is not recommended.

4.1 Introduction

Opioids have been used for medicinal purposes for several thousands of years. The first documented use of opium was in the writings of Theophratus in the third century BC, although it had been used by some of ancient civilizations even earlier. In the early 1800s, the active alkaloids (e.g. morphine, codeine and thebaine) were isolated. Opioids are a mainstay of effective cancer pain management and are increasingly used in the management of other persistent pains. Although their analgesic benefits are well documented in both the scientific literature and the wider public media, so is their potential for abuse, addiction and dependence.

Opioid analgesics occupy steps two and three of the WHO analgesic ladder; those drugs classed as 'weak' opioids (e.g. codeine and dihydrocodeine) being at step two, and 'strong' opioids (e.g. morphine, oxycodone and fentanyl) being at step three. All opioids have a similar mechanism of action. Strong opioids have a linear dose–response curve; however, it is not possible to continue to increase the dose of a weak opioid above a 'ceiling dose' without significantly increasing the incidence of side effects.

'Opiates' are naturally occurring alkaloids from the poppy *Papaver somniferum*, e.g. papaverine, morphine, codeine and thebaine. 'Opioid' refers to all agonists with morphine-like pharmacological activity that can be antagonized by opioid receptor antagonists, e.g. naloxone. In addition to the naturally occurring compounds, the term opioids includes semi-synthetic derivatives (e.g. oxycodone, buprenorphine and hydromorphone) and synthetic compounds (e.g. pethidine, fentanyl and alfentanil).

4.2 **Pharmacology**

In 1973, a family of opioid receptors was identified; endogenous peptides (e.g. enkephalin and endorphin) bound to these receptors with great affinity. Exogenous opioids bound to the same receptors with varying degrees of specificity for the different receptor subtypes. Differential binding to opioid receptor subtypes accounts for the differences in side effects that patients experience with different opioid agonists. Table 4.1 shows the physiological effects of stimulating different opioid receptor subtypes within the central nervous system (CNS) and other systems.

Opioid receptors are examples of G-protein-coupled receptors. Stimulation leads to:

- a reduction in intracellular cyclic adenosine monophosphate (cAMP) by inhibiting the enzyme adenylate cyclase
- the opening of potassium channels thus causing hyperpolarization of the cell membrane
- the inhibition of voltage-gated calcium channels opening thus preventing neurotransmitter release.

Table 4.1 Physiological effects of endogenous opioids	
Receptor	**Physiological response**
μ_1	Supraspinal analgesia
μ_2	Spinal analgesia Respiratory depression Reduced gastrointestinal motility Miosis Euphoria
K	Spinal analgesia Sedation Miosis Dysphoria
δ	Analgesia

4.3 **Opioid tolerance, dependence and addiction**

- Tolerance occurs when identical doses of a drug induce decreasing effects or increasing doses are required to maintain the same effect
- As a result of stopping or reducing prolonged opioid therapy, withdrawal effects may occur which can be physiological (e.g. sweating, tachycardia and diarrhoea) and/or psychological (e.g. craving and agitation)
- Dependence describes the state of requiring a substance or drug to prevent the physiological effects of withdrawal
- Addiction is a syndrome of substance misuse. It includes tolerance and withdrawal, but also loss of control over substance use and relapse after a period of abstinence

  There are relatively little data regarding the rates of these syndromes in patients who have been prescribed opioids for persistent pain. In a retrospective review, despite the trend of increasing therapeutic use of opioids to treat pain there was little evidence of increased health consequences of opioid availability (Joranson et al., 2000).

4.4 **Opioids and non-cancer pain**

The use of opioids to treat pain is common practice in palliative care, but controversy still surrounds their use in patients with chronic non-cancer pain. Over the past 20 years, the use of strong opioids to treat chronic non-cancer pain has increased in the belief that certain patients will derive benefit in analgesia and improvement in function without developing problems of dependence, tolerance and addiction. However, the benefits and risks of long-term opioid therapy need to be carefully monitored. There are very few randomized controlled trials that have studied the long-term effects of opioids in chronic non-cancer pain. Both the practitioner and patient have to exercise careful judgment before embarking on this treatment.

4.4.1 **What is the aim of opioid therapy?**

Opioids should only be used to improve quality of life by managing pain and allowing the patient to optimize their function.

4.4.2 **When should opioids be considered?**

Opioids can only be justified for the treatment of chronic non-cancer pain if:

- other pharmacological methods have failed
- analgesia from opioids is significant and sustained
- the benefits sufficiently outweigh the risks of adverse effects associated with long-term therapy.

4.4.3 **What are the risks associated with long-term opioid therapy?**

Aside from the well-documented adverse effects (see below) of constipation and pruritus, long-term treatment with opioids may be complicated by the development of:

- tolerance (uncommon to see tolerance to the analgesic effect but this would be reflected by increasing analgesic requirements; most patients stabilize on a long-term dose)
- physical dependence (common but usually clinically unimportant providing therapy is not suddenly withdrawn and a modified-release oral or transdermal formulation is used)
- addiction (the compulsive use of opioids to the detriment of the patient's physical, social and psychological well-being)
- endocrine changes (e.g. reduced testosterone, manifesting as fatigue, or reduced libido, infertility)
- immune dysfunction (the clinical implications of this remain unclear).

4.4.4 **Is addiction a problem with long-term opioid use?**

It has been shown in many studies that the risk of developing addictive behaviour on long-term opioid therapy is low. Determining the prevalence of addiction can be difficult as there is some confusion about definitions. It can be mistaken for *pseudo-addiction*, the behaviour that is displayed as a result of physical dependence and poorly controlled pain. There is growing evidence to suggest that the risk of addictive behaviour may be greater than previously thought and further research is warranted.

4.4.5 **What are the recommendations for opioid prescribing?**

- A single practitioner should be responsible for the prescription of opioids
- A treatment plan should be developed and agreed with each patient
- Patients should be informed about adverse effects and risks associated with long-term opioid therapy
- Common side effects should be anticipated and treated, e.g. laxatives and anti-emetics should be co-prescribed
- The use of short-acting opioids regularly for the treatment of chronic non-cancer pain is not recommended. It can precipitate signs of withdrawal between doses which can develop into pseudo-addiction behaviours
- The choice of opioid is made on an individual basis, but modified-release oral or transdermal formulations appear to reduce the risk of apparent behavioural problems

- Previous alcohol abuse or addictive disorders are primary risk factors for problem drug use. Although such patients represent a high risk, they should not be denied therapy. Joint management through a specialist service is recommended
- All pains do not respond to opioids
- A trial of 4–8 weeks therapy may be necessary to determine the response to treatment.

4.5 **Opioid initiation and titration**

In the majority of cases, morphine (see page 37) is the opioid chosen for first-line therapy; alternatives can be used at the discretion of the prescriber. The initial dose of morphine depends on previous opioid exposure and two methods for opioid titration have been adopted for opioid-naive patients:

- An immediate release formulation, 2.5–5 mg every 4 hours is prescribed, with the provision for 'rescue doses' if pain occurs within the 4-hour interval. The rescue dose is one sixth of the total daily morphine dose. The dose of morphine is titrated according to response. When pain control has been achieved and a daily dose of morphine has been established, then a modified release formulation can be introduced. Provision must be made for rescue doses, based on one sixth of the total daily morphine dose
- A modified release formulation, 5–10 mg twice daily is prescribed, with provision for 'rescue doses' if pain occurs within the 4-hour interval. The rescue dose is one sixth of the total daily morphine dose. The modified release dose of morphine is titrated according to response.

Important

- Whatever the choice of opioid, sedation is likely to occur during the titration phase. While tolerance to this effect will develop, patients should be advised that tasks such as driving must be avoided until a stable dose has been achieved
- Nausea and vomiting may also occur, but can be prevented by regular use of an anti-emetic. Tolerance to nausea and vomiting occurs within 5–10 days of initiating treatment after this the anti-emetic can be used as required
- Tolerance to constipation does not occur; regular bowel care and laxative use will be required for as long as the patient receives the opioid.

4.6 **Routes of opioid administration**

Almost all routes of drug delivery have been applied to opioids. Patients who experience inadequate pain relief or intolerable side effects with one opioid often may be successfully treated with another opioid or with the same opioid delivered by a different route (Galer et al., 1992).

4.6.1 **Oral route**

Where possible the oral route should be used for long-term opioid administration for chronic cancer and non-cancer pain. There are marked differences in bioavailability for different opioids. Some opioids undergo a high degree of first pass metabolism (e.g. morphine and fentanyl) resulting in low systemic availability (less than 30%). Other opioids, particularly diamorphine, are quickly converted to active metabolites by plasma esterase enzymes. Several opioids are available in immediate release (given 3–4 hourly) and modified release (given 12 or 24 hourly) formulations. Use of both types of formulation allows analgesia for constant background pain and intermittent (breakthrough or incident) pain.

4.6.2 **Rectal route**

If the oral route is unavailable, then the rectal route may be considered as an alternative; however, systemic absorption can be slow and erratic. Bioavailability may still be low due to first pass metabolism. Increasingly in community settings the subcutaneous route is being used for cancer patients.

4.6.3 **Transdermal route**

Lipophilic opioids, such as buprenorphine and fentanyl, are suited to delivery across the epidermal and dermal layers of the skin. Absorption is slow, so that it can take up to 24 hours after application of the first patch to attain therapeutic plasma concentrations. When considering switching to another opioid following a transdermal formulation it is worth remembering that it will take a similar length of time for plasma concentrations to decline.

4.6.4 **Topical opioids**

See page 87.

4.6.5 **Buccal administration**

Absorption through the epithelium between the gum and cheek has been exploited with the development of oral transmucosal fentanyl citrate (OTFC). Absorption is rapid so these lozenges have been used for the management of breakthrough pain in cancer patients.

4.6.6 **Parenteral opioids**

When patients are unable to take oral medication, opioid administration by the subcutaneous route has become increasingly popular in the management of chronic cancer pain. The intramuscular and intravenous routes are not routinely used in the management of chronic pain. Intramuscular injection of analgesics is often painful and intravenous use is associated with increased side effects, especially respiratory depression and hypotension.

4.6.7 **Spinal opioids**

Opioids may be delivered close to the spinal cord using intrathecal and epidural drug delivery. These 'high tech' delivery methods require suitable equipment and experienced staff. They are costly. They should only be used in specialist centres and when other methods have failed.

4.7 **Morphine**

Morphine is the prototypical strong μ-opioid receptor agonist and is used as the gold standard against which all other opioids are compared. Morphine is recommended as the drug of choice for the management of moderate to severe cancer pain. There is a linear dose–response curve with no ceiling effect; however, the side effects, e.g. sedation and confusion, may preclude reaching optimum analgesia.

4.7.1 **Pharmacology**

When administered orally, morphine undergoes a high degree of first pass metabolism so oral bioavailability is only 20–30%. The elimination half-life of the parent compound is approximately 2 hours; however, the analgesic effects last for around 4 hours. This is probably a result of low lipid solubility, slow uptake in to the CNS and slower elimination from the brain.

The relatively long duration of action may also be associated with formation of at least one pharmacologically active metabolite. Over the past 20 years, there has been great interest in understanding the significance of the two major morphine glucuronide metabolites. Approximately 70% of an oral dose of morphine is metabolized to morphine 3-glucuronide (M3G). A further 10% of a dose is converted to morphine 6-glucuronide (M6G). Other minor metabolites include morphine 3-ethereal sulphate, normorphine and morphine 3,6-diglucuronide. Only 2–10% of the dose is excreted unchanged in urine. The liver is the major organ of morphine metabolism (Hasselstrom *et al.*, 1990), although metabolism has been reported in other tissues including the brain (Sandouk *et al.*, 1991). There is evidence of enterohepatic recycling of morphine (Hasselstrom & Sawe, 1993). The glucuronide metabolites may be deconjugated to morphine by bacteria in the colon after having been excreted in the bile thus allowing re-absorption of the parent compound.

Following oral and intravenous administrations, the plasma concentrations of both glucuronide metabolites exceed that of morphine (Osborne et al., 1990), M6G by twofold and M3G by as much as 20-fold. The elimination half-lives for the glucuronides are much longer than the parent compound and longer than that would be expected for such polar compounds. There is little apparent relationship between morphine and M6G concentrations in plasma and cerebrospinal fluid and pain scores (Somogyi et al., 1993).

M6G is a pharmacologically active metabolite that has a relatively high affinity for μ-opioid receptors. Hence it contributes to the analgesia and side effects of morphine, e.g. respiratory depression, vomiting and sedation (Osborne et al., 1992). The relative analgesic potency of M6G depends on the route of administration. Animal models have suggested M6G:morphine ratios of 2:1 to 650:1; however, it is not clear if this can be translated to humans. The pharmacological effects of M3G are more controversial. M3G shows no affinity for μ- and δ-opioid receptors but intracerebroventricular M3G administration produces allodynia and hyperalgesia (Gong et al., 1992). The overall analgesic effect of morphine is probably the result of a complex interaction of the drug and its two main metabolites.

As the morphine glucuronides are eliminated by urinary excretion, elevated plasma concentrations of M6G have been observed several days after termination of treatment in patients with renal failure (Peterson et al., 1990). Therefore, patients with significant renal impairment need dose reduction to minimize the accumulation of glucuronide metabolites.

4.7.2 **Contraindications and precautions**

- Avoid in patients receiving a MAO-inhibitor.

For the treatment of chronic pain, morphine should be used with caution in the following situations:

- Hypotension
- Asthma/COPD (note that this is not a contraindication)
- Paralytic ileus (assess risk/benefit)
- Empirical dose reduction in patients with hepatic and/or renal impairment may be necessary
- Pregnancy/breastfeeding. Neonates of mothers using opioids during pregnancy may need ventilatory support.

4.7.3 **Adverse effects**

- Nausea/vomiting
- Constipation (prophylactic treatment with a stimulant laxative and faecal softener is often needed)
- Sedation
- Pruritus
- Myoclonus (may indicate overdose)
- Dry mouth
- Sweating
- Vertigo (may add to nausea and vomiting)
- Ureteric or biliary spasm
- Hormonal effects with persistent use (e.g. reduced testosterone concentrations may lead to impotence and infertility)
- Immunosuppression may occur with long-term use.

4.7.4 **Drug interactions**

Pharmacokinetic

- MAO-inhibitors – Morphine should not be started within 2–3 weeks of stopping MAO-inhibitors; MAO-inhibitors should not be started within 2–3 weeks of stopping an opioid.

Pharmacodynamic

Important
• Ensure the opioid dose is reviewed if an adjuvant analgesic is introduced. There may be an opioid-sparing effect.

- Antidepressants—Increased risk of sedation with tricyclic antidepressants.

4.7.5 **Administration**

Important
• Inclusion of brand name on the prescription and dispensing label for morphine preparations is advised for several reasons:
• Dispensing errors have occurred due to confusion between immediate and modified release preparations.
• Patient and carer confusion may lead to potentially serious medication errors.

In the United Kingdom, a wide range of morphine formulations are available commercially and other preparations may be made extemporaneously.

- Immediate release tablets containing 10 mg, 20 mg and 50 mg morphine
- Modified release tablets and capsules containing 5 mg, 10 mg, 15 mg, 30 mg, 60 mg, 100 mg and 200 mg morphine
- Modified release granules containing 20 mg, 30 mg, 60 mg, 100 mg and 200 mg morphine
- Oral solutions containing 10 mg/5 ml and 20 mg/ml morphine
- Suppositories containing 10 mg, 15 mg, 20 mg and 30 mg morphine
- Injection containing 10 mg/ml, 15 mg/ml, 20 mg/ml and 30 mg/ml morphine (1 and 2 ml ampoules).

4.8 Diamorphine

Diamorphine hydrochloride (heroin) is used for medicinal purposes in a relatively small number of countries. It has much greater solubility in water than morphine sulphate and large amounts can be given in a very small volume. There have been supply problems over recent years in the United Kingdom that has significantly reduced its use. It was popular as a spinal drug but its corrosion of the internal workings of some totally implantable pumps now precluded this use.

Diamorphine is more lipophilic than morphine so reaches CNS receptors rapidly. When administered parenterally the effects are due to a metabolite 6-monoacetylmorphine. If given orally diamorphine is a pro-drug for morphine because of deacetylation by plasma esterase enzymes (Brzezinski et al., 1997).

4.9 Codeine

Codeine is a weak μ-opioid receptor agonist on step two of the WHO analgesic ladder; it has 10% of the analgesic potency of morphine.

4.9.1 Pharmacology

Codeine undergoes significant metabolism in the liver, predominately glucuronidation to codeine 6-glucuronide. The analgesic activity of codeine is probably due to cytochrome P-450 mediated O-demethylation to morphine (Yue et al., 1989). Cytochrome CYP2D6 is responsible for this conversion and is subject to genetic polymorphism. Approximately 10% Caucasians and 80% Chinese are unable to metabolize codeine to morphine (Yue et al., 1991). Consequently, some patients may derive no analgesic benefit from codeine.

4.9.2 Contraindications and precautions

See morphine (4.7.2).

4.9.3 Adverse effects

See under morphine (4.7.3).

4.9.4 Drug interactions

See under morphine (4.7.4). Additional pharmacokinetic interactions: Co-administration of CYP2D6 inhibitors may reduce analgesia:

- Paroxetine
- Duloxetine
- Fluoxetine
- Haloperidol
- Levomepromazine.

4.9.5 Administration

Codeine is rarely used as a sole analgesic due to a high incidence of side effects, e.g. nausea and constipation. Combination products containing fixed doses of paracetamol and codeine, such as co-codamol, are available; this makes titration of the individual components difficult.

4.10 Co-proxamol

Co-proxamol (paracetamol 325 mg and dextropropoxyphene 32.5 mg per tablet) has been widely prescribed as an analgesic for many years. However, in January 2005, the MHRA announced a gradual withdrawal of co-proxamol from the UK market because of safety concerns. Dextropropoxyphene may cause fatal apnoea, cardiac arrest or cardiac arrhythmia in overdose with as few as 10–20 tablets. Combination with alcohol or CNS depressant drugs is particularly hazardous. Systematic reviews suggest that co-proxamol is no more effective than paracetamol for acute pain (Li Wan Po & Zhang, 1997). There was significant disquiet at this decision as there are some patients for whom no other analgesic seems to work; an unlicensed product will remain available when other supplies become unavailable.

4.11 Fentanyl

Fentanyl has structural similarity with pethidine. It has a long history of use in anaesthetic and intensive therapy practice as an intravenous analgesic and sedative. Fentanyl is an extremely potent μ-opioid receptor agonist. Owing to a high degree of first pass metabolism it cannot be administered orally. However, it has been formulated for transdermal use in persistent cancer and non-cancer pain, and more recently as OTFC lozenges that may be of use in breakthrough pain.

4.11.1 **Contraindications and precautions**

See morphine (4.7.2).

- Transdermal fentanyl can be used in patients with renal failure as less than 10% is excreted unchanged
- In hepatic disease empirical dose reductions may be necessary
- Increased skin temperature, as the result of a hot bath, or external heat source or fever, may increase absorption from patches
- The transdermal formulation should not be used to treat rapidly changing pain as titration is too slow.

4.11.2 **Adverse effects**

See under morphine (4.7.3).

- Fentanyl tends to be less constipating than morphine (Radbruch *et al.*, 2000) and consequently laxative doses may need to be reviewed
- Transdermal patches may cause local irritation at the site of application
- The lozenge may cause dental caries.

4.11.3 **Drug interactions**

See under morphine (4.7.4).

4.11.4 **Administration**

Transdermal fentanyl patch

As fentanyl is a lipophilic opioid it has suitable physicochemical properties for transdermal delivery. It can take up to 24 hours to reach therapeutic plasma concentrations following application of the first patch as the superficial layers of the skin act as a depot; the drug then becomes slowly available to the systemic circulation. After removal of a patch the elimination half-life is approximately 24 hours compared with three to four hours after intravenous administration (Portenoy *et al.*, 1993). Whilst steady-state plasma concentrations are being established, alternative analgesia (e.g. oral morphine) must be available. There is evidence of efficacy for the management of chronic cancer pain (Ahmedzai & Brooks, 1997), musculoskeletal pain and neuropathic pain (Allan *et al.*, 2001).

Fentanyl is available as both a matrix and reservoir transdermal patch formulation, both available in five different strengths: 12 mcg/hr, 25 mcg/hr, 50 mcg/hr, 75 mcg/hr and 100 mcg/hr. As seen in Table 4.2, each incremental increase equates to a relatively large increase in morphine equivalents per day.

Important

- Inclusion of brand name on the prescription and dispensing label for fentanyl preparations is advised for several reasons:
  - the brands are not interchangeable as therapeutic equivalences cannot be guaranteed
  - patient or carer confusion can lead to potentially serious medication errors

Table 4.2 Recommended conversion between oral morphine and transdermal fentanyl

Oral 24-hour morphine (mg/day)	Transdermal fentanyl (mcg/hr)
<90	25
90–134	37
135–189	50
190–224	62
225–314	75
315–404	100
405–494	125
495–584	150
585–674	175
675–764	200
765–854	225
855–944	250
945–1034	275
1035–1124	300

Important

Transdermal fentanyl patch initiation and titration

- For opioid naive patients, a stable opioid dose should initially be determined using oral morphine as detailed as detailed on page 35
- The response should be assessed after at least 24 hours
- Select patch strength based on this dose using Table 4.2
- The use of short-acting supplemental analgesia (e.g. morphine and oxycodone) is recommended during titration. See Table 4.2 for equivalences
- The application site should be varied, with several days elapsing before applying a patch to the same site
- Although unlicensed, the matrix patch may be cut as the amount released, and hence dose is proportional to the size of the patch. However, patients must not cut reservoir patches as the drug will leak out.

Oral transmucosal fentanyl citrate lozenges

OTFC lozenges are a fentanyl preparation for the treatment of breakthrough pain and are not a long-term alternative for the management of persistent pain. Correct use can provide analgesia within 5–10 minutes; the peak effect is attained in 20–30 minutes (Hanks, 2001).

OTFC is rubbed around the cheek and gum, this allows the lozenge to dissolve in saliva and the fentanyl is absorbed through the buccal mucosa. A further portion of the dose is swallowed and after undergoing first pass metabolism is absorbed into the systemic circulation. Correlation between background opioid requirements and successful OTFC dose is poor (Coluzzi *et al.*, 2001) and so individual titration is required.

4.12 **Hydromorphone**

Hydromorphone is a semi-synthetic strong μ-opioid receptor agonist that is approximately 7.5 times more potent than morphine (Moriarty *et al.*, 1999), although there is marked inter-patient variability in systemic bioavailability. Hydromorphone is metabolized primarily to hydromorphone 3-glucuronide. Accumulation of this metabolite has led to neuroexcitatory side effects (allodynia, myoclonus and seizures) (Smith, 2000). Given intrathecally, it produces less pruritus than morphine.

4.12.1 **Contraindications and precautions**
See under morphine (Section 4.7.2).

4.12.2 **Adverse effects**
See under morphine (4.7.3).

4.12.3 **Drug interactions**
See under morphine (4.7.4).

4.12.4 **Administration**
In the United Kingdom, a range of immediate release and modified release oral formulations are available.

- Immediate release capsules containing 1.3 mg and 2.6 mg hydromorphone
- Modified release capsules (taken 12 hourly) containing 2 mg, 4 mg, 8 mg, 16 mg and 24 mg hydromorphone
- Parenteral formulations are available in some countries; however, only an unlicensed product is available in the United Kingdom.

4.13 **Oxycodone**

Oxycodone has been used for many years in the United States of America in combination with paracetamol or aspirin and because of this it was thought of as a weak opioid. It is a strong opioid agonist with similar analgesic properties to morphine (Glare & Walsh, 1993).

4.13.1 **Pharmacology**

It is a potent μ-receptor agonist that may produce less sedation and hallucinations than morphine in some patients (Maddocks *et al.*, 1996). There is some κ-receptor activity but the clinical effects of oxycodone are that of a μ-receptor agonist. Oral bioavailability of oxycodone is approximately double that of morphine as a result of less first pass metabolism. The equianalgesic ratio of oxycodone: morphine is approximately 1:1.5 (Kalso, 2005), although the manufacturer recommends a ratio of 1:2. Parenteral oxycodone is stated by the manufacturer to be twice as potent as oral, although in practice this is likely to be an overestimate. Oxycodone elimination is impaired in patients with renal failure; dose reduction may be appropriate (Kirvela *et al.*, 1996). Oxycodone has efficacy in chronic cancer (Citron *et al.*, 1998) and non-cancer pain (Watson *et al.*, 2003).

4.13.2 **Contraindications and precautions**

See morphine (4.7.2). In addition, oxycodone is contraindicated in:
- Persistent constipation*
- Pregnancy (and avoid in breastfeeding)
- COPD*
- Moderate to severe hepatic impairment*
- Severe renal impairment*.

4.13.3 **Adverse Effects**

See morphine (4.7.3).

4.13.4 **Drug interactions**

See under morphine (4.7.4). Although metabolism of oxycodone involves the cytochrome system, clinically relevant drug interactions are unlikely to occur. There is a suggestion that the serotonin syndrome may occur with oxycodone and co-administration with SSRIs.

4.13.5 **Administration**

A range of oxycodone formulations are available in the United Kingdom.
- Immediate release capsules containing 5 mg, 10 mg and 20 mg oxycodone
- Modified release tablets containing 5 mg, 10 mg, 20 mg, 40 mg and 80 mg oxycodone

* In palliative care, oxycodone is regularly used in these situations; the prescriber should assess the risk/benefit in each case.

- Oral solution containing 1 mg/ml oxycodone
- Concentrated oral solution containing 10 mg/ml oxycodone
- Injection containing 10 mg/ml oxycodone as 1 ml and 2 ml ampoules.

4.14 Buprenorphine

Buprenorphine is unique among the strong opioids given its partial agonist effect. It has been used to treat chronic moderate to severe cancer and non-cancer pain likely to be sensitive to opioids, especially musculoskeletal pain and neuropathic pain (Sittl et al., 2003).

4.14.1 Pharmacology

Buprenorphine has diverse actions at multiple subtypes of opioid receptor. It is a partial agonist at the μ-opioid receptor agonist, a δ-opioid receptor agonist and a κ-opioid receptor antagonist. The clinical significance of the partial agonist effect at the μ-opioid receptor has been much discussed (Budd & Collett, 2003). There is no evidence for a ceiling dose for analgesia in man, in spite of this being shown for other effects, such as respiratory depression (Dahan et al., 2006).

Buprenorphine does not cause irreversible blockade of opioid receptors, and subsequent use of other opioids is not affected (Walsh et al., 1995). Respiratory depression produced by buprenorphine can be reversed with naloxone, similar to all other opioids, although higher doses may be required. Similar to several other opioids, buprenorphine undergoes extensive first pass metabolism. Buprenorphine is a very lipophilic opioid and has been formulated for transdermal delivery.

4.14.2 Contraindications and precautions

See morphine (4.7.2). In addition, buprenorphine is contraindicated in:
- Pregnancy (and avoid in breastfeeding)
- Myasthenia gravis
- The transdermal formulation should not be used to treat rapidly changing pain; titration is too slow
  The following precautions apply to transdermal buprenorphine:
- Increased skin temperature, either as the result of a hot bath, external heat source or fever, may increase absorption from patches
- Buprenorphine can be used cautiously in patients with renal failure as the pharmacokinetics are unchanged
- Close monitoring is advised in hepatic insufficiency.

4.14.3 **Adverse effects**

See under morphine (4.7.3).

- Transdermal formulations may cause site irritation
- Buprenorphine does not cause the same hormonal effects as other opioids
- Buprenorphine has little immunosuppressive actions.

4.14.4 **Drug interactions**

See under morphine (4.7.4).

- Dose of buprenorphine may need reducing if ketoconazole is co-prescribed
- Carbamazepine may reduce the analgesic benefit of buprenorphine.

4.14.5 **Administration**

Buprenorphine has been available as a tablet for sublingual administration for many years; this formulation is not recommended for chronic pain management. Buprenorphine has been formulated as a matrix patch for transdermal administration. There are two formulations:

- Transdermal matrix patch changed after 96 hours releasing 35 mcg/hr, 52.5 mcg/hr and 70 mcg/hr buprenorphine (Transtec®)
- Transdermal matrix patch changed once weekly releasing 5 mcg/hr, 10 mcg/hr and 20 mcg/hr buprenorphine (Bu-Trans®).

Important

Transdermal buprenorphine patch initiation and titration

- For opioid naive patients, the lowest strength patch should be used initially
- In the case of Bu-Trans®, evaluate response after a minimum of 3 days
- For Transtec®, evaluate response after at least 24 hours
- The use of short-acting supplemental analgesia (e.g. codeine and morphine) is recommended during titration
- Vary the application site with at least 1 week elapsing before applying a patch to the same site
- Although unlicensed, the matrix patch may be cut if necessary as the dose delivered is proportional to the patch size.

4.15 **Methadone**

Methadone is only occasionally used for the treatment of chronic pain because it has a complex pharmacology and dosing schedule. There has been some interest in its use in management of neuropathic pain (Gagnon *et al.*, 2003).

4.15.1 **Pharmacology**

Methadone has a wide range of pharmacological effects. It is a potent agonist at the μ-opioid receptor, an agonist at the δ-opioid receptor, an NMDA (N-methyl-D-asparate) receptor antagonist and it inhibits serotonin pre-synaptic re-uptake.

Methadone has very unusual pharmacokinetic properties that change after multiple dosing. After a single dose, methadone has a high volume of distribution into tissues and biphasic elimination, the half-life in initial phase being 12–24 hours and 55 hours in the secondary phase (Verebely *et al.*, 1975). After prolonged use, more methadone is sequestered in tissues, acting as a depot for continued release in to the systemic circulation, so that the elimination half-life can be up to 80 hours (Sawe, 1986).

4.15.2 **Contraindications and precautions**

See morphine (4.7.2). In addition:

- Use cautiously in patients with risk factors for QT prolongation (e.g. >100 mg/day, heart disease, hepatic impairment, concurrent use of CYP3A4 inhibitors, such as erythromycin—see sub-section Drug interactions below).

4.15.3 **Adverse effects**

See under morphine (4.7.3). In addition:

- Methadone has been used in pregnancy without apparent consequences, but caution is recommended.

4.15.4 **Drug interactions**

See under morphine (4.7.4). There are additional pharmacokinetic interactions:

- Antiretrovirals—Reduced analgesic benefit (e.g. efavirenz, nelfinavir and ritonavir)
- Carbamazepine—Reduced analgesic benefit
- Erythromycin—Increased methadone concentrations and increased risk of QT prolongation
- Fluoxetine—Possible risk of increased methadone concentrations
- Phenytoin—Reduced analgesic benefit.

4.15.5 **Administration**

Methadone titration differs greatly to that of the other oral opioids because of its complex pharmacokinetics. It is rarely initiated for pain as the first-line opioid. A suggested dosage schedule for initiating methadone is shown in Table 4.3.

Methadone is available in a variety of formulations:

- Immediate release tablets containing 5 mg methadone
- Oral solution containing 1 mg/ml methadone
- Oral concentrate containing 10 mg/ml or 20 mg/ml methadone
- Linctus containing 2 mg/5 ml methadone.

Table 4.3 Suggested methadone titration methods

Opioid Naïve

- Start with a regular dose of 2.5–5 mg 12 hourly and 2.5–5 mg every 3 hours as required for pain between regular doses
- Titrate the dose as necessary on a weekly basis, based on the number of as required doses administered within the previous 48 hours
- Do not increase the as required dose in line with the regular dose; continue with 2.5–5 mg
- If the regular dose exceeds 60 mg daily, increase the as required dose to 25% of the 12-hourly dose.

Converting from oral morphine to oral methadone

- Stop morphine
- Give a loading dose of methadone equivalent to 10% of the previous daily morphine dose, up to a maximum of 30 mg, e.g. morphine 120 mg daily, give 12 mg methadone
- If the patient was receiving immediate release morphine, give the methadone 2 hours (pain present) or 4 hours (no pain) after the last dose of morphine
- If the patient was receiving 12-hourly modified release morphine, give the first dose of methadone 6 hours (pain present) or 12 hours (pain free) after the last dose of morphine
- If the patient was receiving 24-hourly modified release morphine, give the first dose of methadone 12 hours (pain present) or 24 hours (pain free) after the last dose of morphine
- Titrate with 3 hourly as required doses of methadone, equivalent to 33% of the loading dose, e.g. 12 mg methadone loading dose, give 4 mg as required
- If analgesia is needed in between the 3 hours, give the as required dose of the previous opioid, e.g. previously taking 120 mg daily of morphine, the as required dose would be 20 mg morphine
- On day 6, total the amount of methadone taken in the previous 48 hours and divide by 4 to give a regular 12-hourly dose. The new as required dose is calculated as 25% of the 12-hourly dose and can be given every 3 hours
- The 12 hourly methadone dose should be reviewed once weekly and any increase should be based on the number of as required doses used.

Key references

Ahmedzai S, Brooks D (1997). Transdermal fentanyl in opioid-naïve cancer pain patients: an open trial using transdermal fentanyl for the treatment of persistent cancer pain in opioid-naïve patients and a group using codeine. *J. Pain Symptom Manage.* **19**: 185–92.

Allan L, Hays H, Jensen N-K, *et al.* (2001). Randomised crossover trial of transdermal fentanyl and sustained release oral morphine for treating persistent non-cancer pain. *Br. Med. J.* **322**: 1154.

Brzezinski MR, Spink BJ, Dean RA, *et al.* (1997). Human liver carboxylesterase hCE-1: binding specificity for cocaine, heroin, and their metabolites and analogs. *Drug Metabol. Dispos.* **25**: 1089–96.

Budd K, Collett BJ (2003). Old dog—new (ma)trix. *Br. J. Anaesth.* **90**: 722–4.

Citron ML, Kaplan R, Parris WC-V (1998). Long-term administration of controlled-release oxycodone tablets for the treatment of cancer pain. *Cancer Invest.* **16**: 562–71.

Coluzzi PH, Schwartzberg L, Conroy Jr JD (2001). Breakthrough cancer pain: a randomized trial comparing oral transmucosal fentanyl citrate (OTFC) and morphine sulfate immediate release (MSIR). *Pain* **91**: 123–30.

Dahan A, Yassen A, Romberg R, *et al.* (2006). Buprenorphine induces ceiling in respiratory depression but not in analgesia. *Br. J. Anaesth.* **96**: 627–32.

Gagnon B, Almahrezi A, Schreier G (2003). Methadone in the treatment of neuropathic pain. *Pain Res. Manage.* **8**: 149–54.

Galer BS, Coyle N, Pasternak GW, Portenoy RK (1992). Individual variability in the response to different opioids: report of five cases. *Pain* **49**: 87–91.

Glare PA, Walsh TD (1993). Dose ranging study of oxycodone for persistent pain in advanced cancer. *J. Clin. Oncol.* **11**: 973–8.

Gong QL, Hedner J, Bjorkman R, Hedner T (1992). Morphine-3-glucuronide may functionally antagonize morphine-6-glucuronide induced antinociception and ventilatory depression in the rat. *Pain* **48**: 249–55.

Hanks G (2001). Oral transmucosal fentanyl citrate for the management of breakthrough pain. *Eur. J. Palliative Care* **8**: 6–9.

Hanks GW, de Conno F, Cherny N, *et al.* (2001). Expert Working Group of the Research Network of the European Association for Palliative Care. *Br. J. Cancer* **84**: 587–92.

Hasselstrom J, Sawe J (1993). Morphine pharmacokinetics and metabolism in humans: enterohepatic cycling and relative contribution of metabolites to active opioid concentrations. *Clin. Pharmacokinet.* **24**: 344–54.

Hasselstrom J, Eriksson S, Perrson A, *et al.* (1990). The metabolism and bioavailability of morphine in patients with severe liver cirrhosis. *Br. J. Clin. Pharmacol.* **29**: 289–97.

Joranson DE, Ryan KM, Gilson AM, Dahl JL (2000). Trends in medical use and abuse of opioid analgesics. *J. Am. Med. Soc.* **283**: 1710–14.

Kalso E (2005). Oxycodone. *J. Pain Symptom Manage.* **29**: S47–S56.

Kirvela M, Lindgren L, Seppala T, Olkkola KT (1996). The pharmacokinetics of oxycodone in uremic patients undergoing renal transplantation. *J. Clin. Anesth.* **8**: 13–18.

Li Wan Po A, Zhang WY (1997). Systematic overview of co-proxamol to assess analgesic effects of addition of dextropropoxyphene to paracetamol. *Br. Med. J.* **315**: 1565–71.

Maddocks I, Somogyi A, Abbott F, *et al.* (1996). Attenuation of morphine-induced delirium in palliative care by substitution with infusion of oxycodone. *J. Pain. Symptom Manage.* **12**: 182–9.

Moriarty M, McDonald CJ, Miller AJ (1999). A randomised crossover comparison of controlled release hydromorphone tablets with controlled release morphine tablets in patients with cancer pain. *J. Clin. Res.* **2**: 1–8.

Osborne R, Joel S, Trew D, Slevin M (1990). Morphine and metabolite behavior after different routes of morphine administration: demonstration of the importance of the active metabolite morphine-6-glucuronide. *Clin. Pharmacol. Ther.* **47**: 12–19.

Osborne R, Thompson P, Joel S, *et al.* (1992). The analgesic activity of morphine-6-glucuronide. *Br. J. Clin. Pharmacol.* **34**: 130–8.

Peterson GM, Randall CTC, Paterson J (1990). Plasma levels of morphine and morphine glucuronides in the treatment of cancer pain: relationship to renal function and route of administration. *Eur. J. Clin. Pharmacol.* **38**: 121–4.

Portenoy RK, Southam MA, Gupta SK, *et al.* (1993). Transdermal fentanyl for cancer pain. Repeated dose pharmacokinetics. *Anesthesiology* **78**: 36–43.

Radbruch L, Sabatowski R, Loick G, *et al.* (2000). Constipation and the use of laxatives: a comparison between transdermal fentanyl and oral morphine. *Palliat. Med.* **14**: 111–19.

Sandouk P, Serrie A, Scherrmann JM, *et al.* (1991). Presence of morphine metabolites in human cerebrospinal fluid after intracerebroventricular administration of morphine. *Eur. J. Drug Metab. Pharmacokinet.* Spec No. **3**: 166–71.

Sawe J (1986). High dose morphine and methadone in cancer patients: clinical pharmacokinetic consideration of oral treatment. *Clin. Pharmacol.* **11**: 87–106.

Sittl R, Griessinger N, Likar R (2003). Analgesic efficacy and tolerability of transdermal buprenorphine in patients with inadequately controlled persistent pain related to cancer and other disorders: a multicenter, randomized, double-blind, placebo-controlled trial. *Clin. Ther.* 25: 150–68.

Smith MT (2000). Neuroexcitatory effects of morphine and hydromorphone: evidence implicating the 3-glucuronide metabolites. *Clin. Exp. Pharmacol. Physiol.* **27**: 524–8.

Somogyi AA, Nation RL, Olweny C, *et al.* (1993). Plasma concentrations and renal clearance of morphine, morphine-3-glucuronide and morphine-6-glucuronide in cancer patients receiving morphine. *Clin. Pharmacokinet.* **24**: 413–20.

Verebely K, Volavka J, Mule S, Resnick R (1975). Methadone in man: pharmacokinetic and excretion studies in acute and persistent treatment. *Clin. Pharmacol. Ther.* **18**: 180–90.

Walsh SL, Preston KL, Bigelow GE, Strizer ML (1995). Acute administration of buprenorphine in humans: partial agonist and blockade effects. *J. Pharmacol. Exp. Ther.* **274**: 361–72.

Watson CPN, Moulin D, Watt-Watson J, *et al.* (2003). Controlled-release oxycodone relieves neuropathic pain: a randomized controlled trial in painful diabetic neuropathy. *Pain* **105**: 71–8.

Yue QY, Svensson JO, Alm C, *et al.* (1989). Codeine O-demethylation co-segregates with polymorphic debrisoquine hydroxylation. *Br. J. Clin. Pharmacol.* **28**: 639–45.

Yue QY, Svensson JO, Sjoqvist F, Sawe J (1991). A comparison of the pharmacokinetics of codeine and its metabolites in healthy Chinese and Caucasian extensive hydroxylators of debrisoquine. *Br. J. Clin. Pharmacol.* **31**: 643–7.

Chapter 5

Antiepileptics

Andrew Dickman and Roger Knaggs

> **Key points**
> - Antiepileptics are effective in a wide range of neuropathic pains
> - Careful titration is required in order to avoid the development of adverse effects
> - Gabapentin and pregabalin are the only antiepileptics licensed for the treatment of neuropathic pain.

5.1 Introduction

Antiepileptics have been used for over 40 years in the management of chronic pain, particularly of a neuropathic type. They reduce neuronal activity and form a diverse group of drugs whose precise mechanism of action is not always completely understood. Currently used drugs are thought to act mainly by three mechanisms shown in Table 5.1. Historically antiepileptics were purported to be of most benefit in neuropathic pain described as 'shooting', they are now known to be effective in a wider range of neuropathic pains involving peripheral and central nervous system (CNS) dysfunction. The largest evidence base is for non-cancer indications, such as diabetic neuropathy and post-herpetic neuralgia, but this has been extrapolated to cancer indications (Berger et al., 2005).

Table 5.1 Mechanism of antiepileptics activity	
Decreasing activity of neuronal sodium channels, enhancing membrane stability	Carbamazepine Phenytoin Lamotrigine Sodium valproate
Decreasing neuronal calcium channel activity	Gabapentin Pregabalin
Increasing synaptic γ-amino butyric acid (GABA) action, either by enhancing GABA activity, inhibiting GABA metabolism or as a GABA agonist	Clonazepam Topiramate Sodium valproate

5.2 Carbamazepine

This was one of the first antiepileptics to be used in neuropathic pain, and is still licensed for the management of trigeminal neuralgia (McQuay et al., 1996; Wiffen et al., 2005a). Its use has declined recently due to its propensity for side effects, drug interactions and the introduction of newer alternatives.

5.2.1 Pharmacology

Carbamazepine inhibits noradrenaline re-uptake and reduces neuronal excitability by a use dependent action on voltage-gated sodium (Na^+) channels (White, 1999). In addition to the activation of descending inhibitory pathways, carbamazepine selectively targets C and Aδ nerve fibres that are firing more frequently than normal (Brodie & Ditcher, 1996). During depolarization, the proportion of Na+ channels in the inactivated state is increased; carbamazepine binds preferentially to channels in this state, thereby reducing the excitability of the neuron. This characteristic permits the attenuation of high frequency discharges without undue alteration of normal functioning. Carbamazepine is relatively well absorbed from the gastrointestinal tract after oral administration and has a bioavailability of approximately 80% (Faigle & Feldman, 1975). The elimination half-life is approximately 30 hours, meaning that it can take several days to reach steady-state plasma concentrations, although this reduces to 15 hours with regular dosing. It is feasible to measure plasma concentrations, similar concentrations being required for managing both trigeminal neuralgia and epilepsy (4–12 mg/L). However, there is substantial variability in drug handling. Carbamazepine is a powerful inducer of hepatic cytochrome P450 enzymes, including those responsible for its own metabolism (Bertilsson et al., 1980); this results in increasing doses being required as a patient is stabilized on the drug, reducing half-life with multiple dosing and many clinically significant interactions with other drugs (see below).

5.2.2 Contraindications and precautions

Carbamazepine is contraindicated with:

- previous bone marrow depression
- acute intermittent porphyria
- MAO-inhibitor; before administering carbamazepine, MAO-inhibitors should be discontinued for a minimum of 2 weeks.

Caution with:

- hepatic or renal impairment
- abrupt withdrawal, as it may lead to seizures
- pregnancy—there is a risk of teratogenesis during the first 12 weeks; folic acid 5 mg daily recommended; vitamin K may need to be given to the mother prior to delivery, as well as the newborn

- breastfeeding—low levels detected in breast milk; unlikely to cause problems
- patients should be warned about driving if affected by drowsiness and dizziness.

5.2.3 Adverse effects

Carbamazepine causes a variety of adverse effects (see manufacturer's SPC for full details) including:

- nausea and vomiting (take with food to overcome)
- oedema, fluid retention, weight increase
- dizziness, ataxia, drowsiness, fatigue (may indicate toxicity)
- blurred vision (may indicate toxicity)
- allergic skin reactions
- haematological disorders (e.g. leucopenia and thrombocytopenia)
- elevated liver enzymes (usually not clinically relevant)
- hyponatraemia.

5.2.4 Drug interactions

Carbamazepine is a potent inducer of the cytochromes CYP3A4 and CYP2C9 creating many pharmacokinetic drug interactions involving metabolism.

- Ciclosporin—Reduced plasma concentrations of ciclosporin
- Clonazepam—Reduced effect of clonazepam
- Corticosteroids—Reduced effect of corticosteroids.

Important

Special considerations

- Haematological disorders, such as leucopenia, thrombocytopenia and aplastic anaemia have occurred with carbamazepine. Patients, relatives and carers should be alerted to the signs of potential haematological problems such as fever, sore throat and easy bruising. If symptoms such as these develop, the patient must consult a doctor and carbamazepine should be discontinued
- Liver function tests should be performed prior to treatment and periodically throughout therapy. Raised liver enzymes, such as γGT and ALP, can occur; these are not an indication to stop treatment. If liver damage is suspected, carbamazepine dosing should be temporarily suspended
- Skin reactions such as mild erythema are usually transient and resolve within days or weeks. If a rash becomes more severe, carbamazepine should be withdrawn immediately.
- Hyponatraemia is more common in the elderly and can present as drowsiness, confusion, or convulsions. Concurrent use of an antidepressant may increase this risk.

- Haloperidol—Reduced plasma concentrations of haloperidol
- Methadone—Reduced plasma concentrations of methadone
- Mirtazapine—Reduced plasma concentrations of mirtazapine
- Oestrogens—Reduced plasma concentrations of oestrogens; risk of contraception failure
- Progestogens—Reduced plasma concentrations of progestogens; risk of contraception failure.

There are several pharmacodynamic interactions involving carbamazepine and drugs that lower the seizure threshold which can affect its control of epilepsy, e.g. interaction with tricyclic antidepressants and antipsychotics. Alcohol enhances the CNS effects of carbamazepine.

5.2.5 **Administration**

Carbamazepine is available as immediate and modified release tablets, chewable tablets, liquid and suppositories (125 mg suppositories are equivalent to 100 mg tablets). Carbamazepine is indicated for the treatment of trigeminal neuralgia, although it is often used for other causes of neuropathic pain. It is a unique drug in that it auto-induces its own metabolism. Consequently, carbamazepine must be started at a low dose and gradually increased according to response. Typically, an initial dose of 100 mg twice daily is introduced and increased gradually over 5–10 days in increments of 100–200 mg until pain is controlled, or a maximum daily dose of 1600 mg is achieved. The usual maintenance dose is 200 mg 3–4 times daily. Long-term carbamazepine therapy must not be suddenly withdrawn due to the risk of seizures.

5.3 **Gabapentin**

Gabapentin is a widely prescribed antiepileptic for the treatment of chronic pain due to the improved tolerability and lack of drug interactions compared with earlier antiepileptics. Gabapentin is an effective treatment for peripheral neuropathic pain, although carbamazepine may be a more effective option (Wiffen et al., 2005b).

5.3.1 **Pharmacology**

Gabapentin was originally developed as an agonist of the $GABA_A$ receptor, but was subsequently found to be devoid of GABA effects. The analgesic benefit of gabapentin is due to its affinity for the $\alpha_2\delta$ subunit of voltage-dependent calcium channels (Gee et al., 1996). Gabapentin binds to the $\alpha_2\delta$ subunit, effectively closing the channel and preventing the release of neurotransmitters and modulators. In animal models, it may have anti-nociceptive effects in inflammatory pain (Stanfa et al., 1997). Early clinical experience suggests that its combination with opioids may be of additional benefit for the treatment of neuropathic pain (Keskinbora *et al.*, 2007). Gabapentin is readily absorbed after oral administration; however, the mechanism of absorption is saturable as it is dependent on utilizing the amino acid carrier system. Therefore, increasing the dose does not proportionally increase the amount absorbed. Bioavailability of gabapentin after oral administration is approximately 60% and the plasma elimination half-life is approximately 6 hours (Cornstock *et al.*, 1990); this necessitates administration three times a day. Gabapentin is largely excreted unchanged in the urine, so dose adjustment is needed in renal impairment.

5.3.2 Contraindications and precautions

- Avoid sudden withdrawal. Discontinue gradually over at least 1 week in order to reduce effects such as nausea, vomiting, anxiety and insomnia
- Caution in renal impairment—dosage adjustments may be necessary (see below)
- If affected by drowsiness and dizziness, patients should be warned about driving
- Caution in pregnancy and breastfeeding. Human data are lacking, so avoid unless the benefits to the mother outweigh the potential risks to the foetus/baby.

5.3.3 Adverse effects

Gabapentin is generally well-tolerated with few serious adverse effects if titration is started at low dose and proceeds slowly. Most of the adverse effects described below are usually dose-related, e.g.

- drowsiness
- dizziness
- nausea and vomiting
- diarrhoea
- asthenia
- tremor
- oedema
- loss if libido
- pancreatitis (withdraw gabapentin)
- peripheral oedema.

5.3.4 Drug interactions

Gabapentin is one of the few antiepileptics that lack clinically relevant drug interactions, mainly due to no significant hepatic metabolism and low protein binding. The vast majority of drug interactions are pharmacodynamic and can be anticipated, e.g. co-prescription with a strong opioid increases the risk of CNS depression.

5.3.5 **Administration**

Gabapentin is indicated for the treatment of peripheral neuropathic pain. It is currently only available as tablets and capsules. The capsules can be opened if necessary, prior to administration, and given in water or fruit juice. The licensed starting dosage schedule is shown in Table 5.2. Many patients, particularly the elderly or those with cancer, will be unable to tolerate this regimen; for these patients, a more cautious approach is suggested as shown in Table 5.2. Whichever strategy is adopted, adverse effects are more common around the time of dose escalation but usually resolve in a few weeks. Slower titration may be preferred in the elderly or cancer population, although it may take longer to appreciate the therapeutic benefit. Dose adjustments are also necessary for patients in renal failure or undergoing haemodialysis and are shown in Tables 5.3 and 5.4, respectively.

Table 5.2 Dosage schedules for gabapentin			
Licensed		**Suggested**	
Day 1	300 mg nocte	Day 1	100 mg nocte
Day 2	300 mg twice daily	Day 2	100 mg twice daily
Day 3	300 mg three times daily	Day 3	100 mg three times daily
Increase by 300 mg daily according to response up to a maximum of 1.2 g three times daily		Increase by 100 mg three times daily every 2 days as needed to a maximum of 1.2 g three times daily	

Table 5.3 Recommended gabapentin dosage adjustments based on renal function	
Creatinine clearance (ml/min)	**Maximum dose**
≥80	1200 mg three times daily
50–79	600 mg three times daily
30–49	300 mg three times daily
15–29	300 mg once daily
<15	300 mg alternate days to once daily
Adjust starting dose as necessary.	

Table 5.4 Haemodialysis dosage adjustments for gabapentin	
Anuric patients	**Renally impaired patients**
Initial loading dose of 300–400 mg, then 200–300 mg of gabapentin following each 4 hours of haemodialysis. On dialysis-free days, there should be no treatment with gabapentin.	Dose as per Table 5.3 based on creatinine clearance. An additional 200–300 mg dose following each 4-hour haemodialysis treatment is recommended.

5.4 **Pregabalin**

Pregabalin is an antiepileptic with very similar properties to gabapentin. It is relatively well-tolerated and lacks clinically relevant drug interactions. It has been shown to be effective for neuropathic pain and has anxiolytic and sleep-modulating effects (Gajraj, 2005).

5.4.1 **Pharmacology**

Pregabalin was originally developed as a GABA analogue for the treatment of epilepsy, but like gabapentin, it is inactive at GABA receptors and has no GABA-like activity. The precise mechanism of action remains uncertain, but pregabalin does interact with the same binding site as gabapentin ($\alpha_2\delta$ subunit of the voltage-dependent calcium channel), with a binding affinity six times that of gabapentin (Tremont Lukats $et\ al.$, 2000; Selak, 2001). Binding to the $\alpha_2\delta$ subunit effectively closes the channel and prevents the release of neurotransmitters and modulators. Pregabalin has a linear pharmacokinetic profile. Its mean bioavailability is greater than 90% (Bialer $et\ al.$, 2001) and is independent of dose; this is a major difference to gabapentin. Elimination half-life of pregabalin is also longer, ranging from 5.5 to 6.7 hours (published pharmacokinetic data). Pregabalin is excreted by the kidneys, with 98% of an administered dose being excreted unchanged in urine, so dose adjustment is required in renal impairment (see page 60).

5.4.2 **Contraindications and precautions**

Avoid sudden withdrawal. Discontinue gradually over at least 1 week to avoid adverse effects such as nausea, vomiting, anxiety and insomnia. These withdrawal effects have been reported even after short-term use.

- Caution in renal impairment—dosage adjustments may be necessary (see below)
- Use with caution in patients with congestive heart failure
- If affected by drowsiness and dizziness, patients should be warned about driving
- Caution in pregnancy and breastfeeding. Human data are lacking, so avoid unless the benefits to the mother outweigh the potential risks to the foetus/baby.

5.4.3 **Adverse effects**

Pregabalin is generally well-tolerated with mainly dose-dependent adverse effects that are mild to moderate. They include:

- weight gain
- dizziness
- drowsiness
- peripheral oedema
- visual disturbances.

5.4.4 **Drug Interactions**

Pregabalin is one of the few antiepileptics that lack clinically relevant drug interactions, mainly due to no significant hepatic metabolism and low protein binding. The vast majority of drug interactions are pharmacodynamic and can be anticipated, e.g. co-prescription with a strong opioid can increase the risk of CNS depression.

5.4.5 **Administration**

Pregabalin is indicated for the treatment of central and peripheral neuropathic pains. It is also indicated for the treatment of anxiety. Pregabalin is currently only available as capsules which may be opened, if necessary, prior to use and given in water or fruit juice. The licensed dosing schedule is shown in Table 5.5. As with gabapentin, this may be poorly tolerated by elderly patients or those with cancer, and for these patients, a more cautious titration is advised, as in Table 5.5. Whichever strategy is adopted, adverse effects are more common around the time of dose escalation but usually resolve in a few weeks. The slower titration may be preferred in the elderly or cancer population, although it may take longer to appreciate the therapeutic benefit. Dose adjustments are also necessary for patients in renal failure or undergoing haemodialysis and are shown in Table 5.6.

Table 5.5 Dosage schedules for pregabalin			
Licensed		Suggested	
Day 1	75 mg twice daily	Day 1	25 mg nocte
Day 3–7	150 mg twice daily	Day 2	25 mg twice daily
Day 10–14	300 mg twice daily	Day 7	75 mg twice daily
Increase dose according to response. Max dose 600 mg/day. Dose can be given three times daily if needed		Increase dose by 25 mg twice daily every 2 days as needed to a maximum of 600 mg daily	

Table 5.6 Recommended pregabalin dosage adjustments based on renal function	
Creatinine clearance (ml/min)	Maximum dose
≥60	300 mg twice daily
≥30–<60	150 mg twice daily
≥15–<30	75 mg twice daily or 150 mg once daily
<15	75 mg once daily
Adjust starting dose as necessary. A supplementary dose (maximum 100 mg/day) should be given immediately following every 4-hour haemodialysis treatment.	

5.5 **Other antiepileptic drugs**

Many other antiepileptic drugs, including topiramate, clonazepam, tiagabine and levetiracetam, have been used in the management of chronic pain, although only lamotrigine (Vestergaard *et al.*, 2001) and phenytoin (McCleane, 1999), in addition to carbamazepine, gabapentin and pregabalin, have been the subject of randomized double blind clinical trials.

Clonazepam appears to be a popular choice in palliative care and anecdotal evidence suggests that it is well-tolerated and effective for neuropathic pain. Its mode of action probably involves GABA modulation. It is available as tablets, oral solution and injection. Although unlicensed, clonazepam can be administered via continuous subcutaneous infusion.

Lamotrigine was originally marketed as an adjunct treatment for partial seizures. It blocks voltage-dependent sodium channels and inhibits the release of the excitatory neurotransmitter glutamate (Perucca, 1993). Up to 10% patients may develop a rash, which very occasionally may develop into Stevens-Johnson syndrome or toxic epidermal necrolysis. A recent review concluded that lamotrigine is unlikely to be of benefit in neuropathic pain (Wiffen & Rees, 2007).

Phenytoin stabilizes neuronal cells by blocking sodium channels and inhibits pre-synaptic glutamate release at higher concentrations. Side effects (e.g. gingival hyperplasia, hair thickening and many CNS side effects) and a narrow therapeutic index have limited its routine use in pain management.

Key references

Berger A, Dukes E, Mercadante S, Oster G (2005). Use of anticonvulsants and tricyclic antidepressants in cancer patients with neuropathic pain. *Eur. J. Cancer Care* **15**: 138–45.

Bertilsson L, Hojer B, Tybring G, *et al.* (1980). Autoinduction of carbamazepine metabolism in children. *Clin. Pharamacol. Ther.* **27**: 83.

Bialer M, Johannessen SI, Kupferberg HJ, *et al.* (2001). Progress report on new anticonvulsant drugs: a summary of the fifth Eilat conference (EILAT V). *Epilepsy Res.* **43**: 11–58.

Brodie MJ, Ditcher MA (1996). Anti-convulsant drugs. *New Eng. J. Med.* **334**: 168–75.

Cornstock TJ, Sica DA, Bockbrader HN, *et al.* (1990). Gabapentin pharmacokinetics in subjects with various degrees of renal impairment. *J. Clin. Pharmacol.* **30**: 862.

Faigle JW, Feldman KF (1975). Pharmacokinetic data of carbamazepine and its major metabolites in man. In H Schneider, D Janz, C Gardner-Thorpe, H Meinardi, AL Shervin (eds), *Clinical Pharmacology of Anticonvulsant Drugs* (pp. 159–65). Springer-Verlag, Berlin.

Gajraj NM (2005). Pregabalin for pain management. *Pain Pract.* **5**: 95–102.

Gee NS, Brown JP, Dissanayake VU, *et al.* (1996). The novel anticonvulsant drug, gabapentin (Neurontin), binds to the alpha-2delta subunit of the calcium channel. *J. Biol. Chem.* **271**: 5768–76.

Keskinbora K, Pekel AF, Aydinli I (2007). Gabapentin and an opioid combination versus opioid alone for the management of neuropathic cancer pain: a randomized open trial. *J. Pain Symptom Manage.* **34**: 183–9.

McCleane GJ (1999). Intravenous infusion of phenytoin relieves neuropathic pain: a randomized, double-blinded, placebo-controlled, crossover study. *Anesth. Analg.* **89**: 985–988.

McQuay H, Carroll D, Jadad AR, *et al.* (1996). Anticonvulsant drugs for the management of pain: a systematic review. *Br. Med. J.* **311**: 1047.

Perucca E (1993). The clinical pharmacology of the new anticonvulsant drugs. *Pharmacol. Res.* **28**: 89–106.

Selak I (2001). Pregabalin. *Curr. Opin. Investig. Drugs* **2**: 828.

Stanfa LC, Singh L, Williams RG, Dickenson AH (1997). Gabapentin, ineffective in normal rats, markedly reduces C-fibre evoked responses after inflammation. *Neuro report* **8**: 587.

Tremont Lukats IW, Megeff C, Backonja MM (2000). Anticonvulsants for neuropathic pain syndromes: mechanisms of action and place in therapy. *Drugs* **60**: 1029–52.

Vestergaard K, Andersen G, Gottrup H, *et al.* (2001). Lamotrigine for central poststroke pain; a randomized controlled trial. *Neurology* **56**: 184–90.

White HS (1999). Comparative anticonvulsant and mechanistic profile of the established and newer anticonvulsant drugs. *Epilepsia* **40** (Suppl 5): S2–S10.

Wiffen PJ, Rees J (2007). Lamotrigine for acute and chronic pain. *Cochrane Database Syst. Rev.* **2**: CD006044.

Wiffen PJ, McQuay HJ, Moore RA (2005a). Carbamazepine for acute and chronic pain. *Cochrane Database Syst. Rev.* **3**: CD005451.

Wiffen PJ, McQuay HJ, Edwards JE, Moore RA (2005b). Gabapentin for acute and chronic pain. *Cochrane Database Syst. Rev.* **3**: CD005452.

Chapter 6

Antidepressants

Andrew Dickman and Roger Knaggs

Key points

- Not all antidepressants are effective for the management of neuropathic pain
- Tricyclic antidepressants, such as amitriptyline, are the gold standard to which others are compared, while SSRIs appear ineffective
- Of the newer agents, only duloxetine has a license for pain management, specifically for diabetic neuropathy.

6.1 Introduction

Antidepressants have been used for several decades in the treatment of chronic pain. The largest evidence base is for non-cancer indications, such as diabetic neuropathy and post-herpetic neuralgia (Sindrup et al., 2005), but this evidence has been extrapolated to cancer pain (Berger et al., 2005). Most studies have used tricyclic antidepressants (TCAs) e.g. amitriptyline, desipramine, which increase the amount of monoamine neurotransmitters (noradrenaline and serotonin (5-HT)) in the central nervous system (CNS) by inhibiting the re-uptake of neurotransmitter from the synaptic cleft. The prototype antidepressant drug used in pain management is amitriptyline, but many other antidepressants with more novel mechanisms of action have become available over more recent years, e.g. selective serotonin re-uptake inhibitors (SSRIs), e.g. fluoxetine citalopram, paroxetine and sertraline. SSRIs appear to be less effective than TCAs in producing analgesia and will not be discussed further. Monoamine oxidase (MAO) inhibitors are rarely used as analgesics. Several new antidepressants, e.g. venlafaxine, duloxetine and mirtazapine, that selectively increase a range of amine neurotransmitters have been marketed; early clinical trial results suggest a possible greater role for some of these drugs in pain management.

6.2 **Tricyclic antidepressants**

TCAs have complex pharmacological effects; some explain their pharmacological benefits and others determine their side effects. Amitriptyline is the most commonly studied TCA; its use is associated with many side effects that often prevent patients reaching therapeutic doses. Patients may experience adverse effects within hours of taking the first dose but the analgesic effect becomes apparent much more slowly (Botney et al., 1983; Max et al., 1987).

6.2.1 **Pharmacology**

Noradrenaline and serotonin, with endogenous opioids and γ-amino butyric acid (GABA), modulate the activity of descending inhibitory pain pathways from the brainstem and midbrain; they act in the dorsal horn of the spinal cord and in other areas in the CNS (Basbaum & Fields, 1984). Antidepressants modulate spinal cord pain transmission by inhibiting the re-uptake of noradrenaline and serotonin. Antidepressants may also improve mood by their conventional antidepressant action in patients with chronic pain. In vitro data suggest that some antidepressants may block sodium and calcium channels (Song et al., 2000) and are NMDA (N-methyl-D-aspartate) receptor antagonists (Eisenach & Gebhart, 1995). The receptor affinity and pharmacological profile of commonly used antidepressants are summarized in Table 6.1.

TCAs can be divided into tertiary amines and their N-demethylated, secondary amine derivatives. Tertiary TCAs include amitriptyline, imipramine and clomipramine. Secondary TCAs include nortriptyline and desipramine. There is limited evidence that secondary amine TCAs have fewer anticholinergic, antihistaminergic and $\alpha 1$ adrenoceptor antagonist side effects compared with tertiary amines.

TCAs should be given orally; as they all have a long elimination half-life, once daily dosing is sufficient. They are usually taken approximately 2 hours before bed because of their sedative effects. The relationship between plasma concentrations and analgesic response is not clear; it appears that a critical plasma concentration must be achieved for efficacy. Routine plasma monitoring is not warranted.

6.2.2 **Contraindications and precautions**

TCAs are contraindicated in patients with:
- recent myocardial infarction
- severe liver disease
- porphyria
- MAO-inhibitor co-administration (concurrent or within 2 weeks of taking; see Drug Interactions, section 6.2.4)
  TCAs should be used cautiously in:
- the elderly where the incidence of adverse effects is high.

Table 6.1 Pharmacological profile of antidepressants used in pain management

		TCA		SSRI	SNRI
		Amitriptyline Clomipramine	Nortriptyline Desipramine	Fluoxetine Paroxetine Citalopram	Venlafaxine Duloxetine
Reuptake inhibition	Noradrenaline	++	++	−	++
	Serotonin	+	−	++	+
Receptor blockade	Muscarinic acetylcholine	++	++	−	−
	H_1-histaminergic	++	++	−	−
	α-Adrenergic	+	+	−	
	NMDA	+	+	−	−
Ion channel blockade	Sodium channels	+	+	±/?	±
	Calcium channels	+	+	?	?

TCA–tricyclic antidepressant drug; SSRI–selective serotonin reuptake inhibitor; SNRI–Selective noradrenaline reuptake inhibitor.

- patients with severe depression/suicide risk; the therapeutic index (i.e. difference between therapeutic and toxic plasma concentrations) is small and TCAs in overdose may be fatal
- patients with epilepsy or history of convulsions (TCAs lower seizure threshold)
- patients at risk of urinary retention or with prostate hypertrophy (TCAs can precipitate urinary retention)
- patients in whom sedation would interfere with work or driving; a newer TCA with less antimuscarinic side effects (e.g. lofepramine) or SSRI may be more appropriate
- patients with low plasma sodium, especially the elderly. All types of antidepressant lower plasma sodium concentrations. Hyponatraemia should be considered in patients who develop drowsiness, confusion or convulsions when taking an antidepressant
- patients with glaucoma
- pregnancy as limited safety data are available
- breastfeeding as significant concentrations are present in breast milk.

TCAs must not be stopped abruptly, as sleep disturbance, irritability and other less specific CNS effects have been described. To minimize these effects the dose should be reduced gradually over a period of weeks or months, depending on the length of time that a patient has been taking the drug.

6.2.3 **Adverse effects**

The most common and troublesome side effects are associated with non-specific blockade of H_1 histamine receptors and muscarinic acetylcholine receptors. Typical adverse effects include:

- dry mouth—use of saliva substitutes/sucking sweets may help
- blurred vision—a problem if patients drive or operate machinery; once the dose has been stabilized tolerance to this effect develops
- urinary retention
- constipation
- sexual dysfunction
- increased intraocular pressure
- sedation and drowsiness
- confusion
- nightmares
- arrhythmias, syncope and postural hypotension
- reversible alteration in liver enzymes
- hepatitis
- hyponatraemia (may present as drowsiness, confusion or convulsions).

Important

Patients should be warned about potential adverse effects before starting TCAs and informed that these should improve as tolerance develops. Starting with a low dose and gradual titration may reduce the incidence of anticholinergic effects.

6.2.4 **Drug interactions**

Pharmacokinetic

- Antiepileptics—metabolism of TCA increased by barbiturates, carbamazepine and phenytoin (reduced effect)
- Rifampicin—metabolism of TCA increased (reduced effect)
- SSRIs—plasma levels of TCAs may be increased by paroxetine and fluoxetine
- Warfarin—clotting problems; INR may be increased or reduced by TCAs.

Pharmacodynamic

- Alcohol—increased sedative effect
- Anti-arrhythmics—increased risk of arrhythmias

- Antiepileptics—antiepileptic effect antagonized as seizure threshold lowered; increased risk of sedation
- Antipsychotics—increased risk of arrhythmias and anticholinergic effects; increased risk of sedation
- Clonidine—increased risk of hypotension
- MAO-inhibitors—TCAs should not be started within 2–3 weeks of stopping MAO-inhibitors; MAO-inhibitors should not be started within 2–3 weeks of stopping a TCA
- Opioids—increased sedative effect
- SSRIs—increased risk of serotonin syndrome
- Tramadol—increased risk of CNS toxicity; possibly serotonin syndrome.

6.2.5 **Administration**

TCAs are available as tablets, capsules and oral liquids; there are no parenteral formulations. None of the TCAs are licensed for the treatment of neuropathic pain. A low TCA starting dose may reduce adverse effects, e.g. amitriptyline 5–10 mg at night; this should be titrated upwards over a period of weeks and generally a dose of 50–75 mg is required to produce analgesia. Even at this dose there is a significant drop-out rate from clinical trials due to side effects.

6.3 **Other antidepressants**

Venlafaxine is a selective serotonin and noradrenaline re-uptake inhibitor (SNRI). Venlafaxine increases the synaptic concentration of the monoamine neurotransmitters, noradrenaline and serotonin, in a manner similar to TCAs. It does not have the same effects on H_1 histamine receptors, α_1-adrenoceptors and muscarinic acetylcholine receptors. Therefore, some of the most bothersome side effects associated with TCA therapy are reduced with an SNRI. Adverse effects of venlafaxine include nausea, constipation, sedation, dry mouth, sexual dysfunction and dizziness. There are no randomized controlled trials that directly compare venlafaxine to amitriptyline, although there is evidence of analgesic benefit with venlafaxine in patients with diabetic neuropathy, fibromyalgia, headache and several other chronic pain conditions (Tasmuth et al., 2002).

67

Important
Venlafaxine must not be stopped abruptly, as sleep disturbance, headache, nausea, vomiting and other less specific CNS effects have been described. To minimize these effects, the dose should be reduced gradually over a period of weeks.

Duloxetine a more recently introduced SNRI, appears to have similar analgesic efficacy to venlafaxine in standard models of neuropathic pain, e.g. diabetic neuropathy (Goldstein *et al.*, 2005) and other pain conditions, e.g. fibromyalgia (Arnold *et al.*, 2005). It has similar adverse effects to venlafaxine. A withdrawal reaction has not been described for duloxetine, but it is prudent to withdraw therapy over several weeks. Further evidence is required for the analgesic effects of these SNRIs before widespread use is acceptable.

Key references

Arnold LM, Rosen A, Pritchett YL, D'Souza DN, *et al.* (2005). A randomized, placebo-controlled trial of duloxetine in the treatment of women with fibromyalgia with or without major depressive disorder. *Pain* **119**: 5–15.

Basbaum AI, Fields HL (1984). Endogenous pain control systems: brain stem spinal pathways and endorphin circuitry. *Ann. Rev. Neurosci.* **7**: 309–38.

Berger A, Dukes E, Mercadante S, Oster G (2005). Use of antiepileptics and tricyclic antidepressants in cancer patients with neuropathic pain. *Eur. J. Cancer Care* **15**: 138–45.

Botney M, Fields HC (1983). Amitriptyline potentiates morphine analgesia by direct action on the central nervous system. *Ann. Neuro.* **13**: 160–4.

Eisenach JC, Gebhart GF (1995). Intrathecal amitriptyline acts an N-methyl-D-asparate receptor antagonist in the presence of inflammatory hyperalgesia in rats. *Anesthesiol.* **83**: 1046–54.

Goldstein DJ, Lu Y, Dteke MJ, *et al.* (2005). Duloxetine *vs* placebo in patients with painful diabetic neuropathy. *Pain* **116**: 109–18.

Max MB, Culnane M, Schafer SC, *et al.* (1987). Amitriptyline relieves diabetic neuropathy pain in patients with normal and depressed mood. *Neurology* **37**: 589–96.

Sindrup SH, Otto M, Finnerup NB, *et al.* (2005). Antidepressants in the treatment of neuropathic pain. *Pharmacol. Toxicol.* **96**: 399–409.

Song JH, Ham SS, Shin YK, *et al.* (2000). Amitriptyline modulation of Na$^+$ channels in rat dorsal route ganglion neurons. *Eur. J. Pharmacol.* **401**: 297–305.

Tasmuth T, Hartel B, Kalso E (2002). Venlafaxine in neuropathic pain following treatment of breast cancer. *Eur. J. Pain* **6**: 17–24.

Chapter 7

Miscellaneous analgesics

Andrew Dickman and Roger Knaggs

> **Key points**
> - A wide range of other pharmacological options are available for the management of chronic pain
> - Topical formulations offer a novel, less toxic method of drug administration
> - Most of these drugs, with the notable exception of the lidocaine plaster, are not considered first-line choices.

7.1 Anti-arrhythmics

Lidocaine and mexiletine are sodium channel blockers and have membrane-stabilizing properties. Flecainide is similar to mexiletine, but due to reports of increased mortality, its use has declined. Topical lidocaine is discussed elsewhere (see section 7.7). Intravenous lidocaine has been shown to have analgesic benefit in a variety of chronic pain syndromes, particularly peripheral neuropathic pain (Challapalli et al., 2005; Tremont-Lukats et al., 2006), although studies of cancer-related neuropathic pain showed negative results (Ellemann et al., 1989; Bruera et al., 1992). There may be a prolonged analgesic effect after a single intravenous lidocaine infusion. If benefit is achieved, then therapy may be continued either with a subcutaneous infusion or possibly with oral mexiletine. However, the subsequent benefit of oral mexiletine after successful intravenous lidocaine use has not been established for pain. Mexiletine has been successfully used as the initial anti-arrhythmic therapy in a variety of peripheral neuropathic pains (Sloan, 1999; Challapalli et al., 2005), although there have been no controlled trials in cancer-related neuropathic pain.

7.1.1 Pharmacology

Lidocaine and mexiletine are structurally similar drugs and their main indication for use is cardiac arrhythmias. Local anaesthetics block sodium channels thereby reducing the excitability of the neuron and reducing pain transmission; this explains the analgesic effect of topically applied and locally instilled lidocaine. The systemic actions of lidocaine and mexiletine are not completely understood. It is believed that, as with topical and local use, the systemic action involves the selective blockade of hyperexcitable neurons since these drugs will only work when the sodium channel is open.

Lidocaine is rapidly metabolized by the liver via cytochrome CYP3A4. The metabolites have similar pharmacology to lidocaine, but are less potent. Approximately 90% of administered lidocaine is excreted by the kidneys as metabolites with approximately 10% being excreted unchanged.

Mexiletine is well-absorbed orally and it is metabolized by the hepatic isozymes CYP2D6 and CYP1A2 to mainly inactive compounds; small amounts of a weakly acting metabolite are produced. The metabolites and unchanged drug are excreted by the kidneys.

7.1.2 Contraindications and precautions

Lidocaine

- Contraindicated for patients with hypersensitivity to amide local anaesthetics
- Contraindicated in porphyria
- Metabolic disturbances, such as hypokalaemia and hypoxia, should be corrected before commencing lidocaine
- Avoid in pregnancy and breastfeeding unless benefits outweigh risks.

Mexiletine

- Contraindicated in the first 3 months after a myocardial infarction
- Avoid in patients with a known hypersensitivity to amide local anaesthetics
- Avoid in pregnancy and breastfeeding.

Given the hepatic metabolism, both drugs should be used cautiously in patients with significant hepatic impairment and individual dose titration is recommended. Dose reduction may be necessary in severe renal impairment. Both drugs should be used with caution in patients with sinus node dysfunction, conduction defects, bradycardia, hypotension or cardiac failure. Mexiletine should be tapered upon discontinuation, rather than abruptly stopped.

7.1.3 Adverse effects

Adverse effects experienced with lidocaine are generally dose related. They include:

- light-headedness
- hypotension
- bradycardia
- drowsiness
- dizziness
- convulsions
- cardiac arrest
- respiratory arrest.

The main adverse effects of mexiletine are dose related and include:

- nausea and vomiting (often signalling the end of a therapeutic trial)
- drowsiness
- dizziness
- blurred vision
- hypotension
- sinus bradycardia
- atrial fibrillation and torsade de pointes
- convulsions.

7.1.4 Drug interactions

Pharmacokinetic

- Given the involvement of the cytochrome system, drugs that influence the activity of CYP3A4 and CYP2D6/CYP1A2 should be used carefully with lidocaine and mexiletine, respectively
- Opioids and anti-cholinergic drugs delay the absorption of mexiletine.

Pharmacodynamic

- There is an additive risk of myocardial depression when lidocaine or mexiletine are used with other anti-arrhythmics.

7.1.5 Administration

Neither drug has a licensed indication for the treatment of pain, although there is ample clinical experience. Lidocaine is typically infused over 30 minutes within the range of 1–5 mg/kg/day, starting at the lower range for frail or elderly patients. It is recommended that an ECG is performed before starting lidocaine, or increasing the dose and the patient should be carefully monitored throughout the infusion and for a short time afterwards.

Mexiletine is administered at doses lower than those used for arrhythmias. A dose of 50 mg three times daily is used initially, increasing to a maximum of 900 mg/day.

7.2 Bisphosphonates

Bisphosphonates are analogues of inorganic pyrophosphate that work by inhibiting osteoclast activity. They reduce skeletal complications of bone metastases, and also have an analgesic effect which should be apparent within 14 days of initiating treatment (Wong & Wiffen, 2002; Yuen et al., 2006; Cralow & Tripathy, 2007). Bisphosphonates have also shown benefits in other painful conditions such as CRPS and Paget's disease (Hasking, 2006; Eisenberg et al., 2007).

7.2.1 Pharmacology

Inorganic pyrophosphate and bisphosphonates have the chemical structures shown in Figure 7.1. Note the P–O–P backbone of pyrophosphate and the similar P–C–P backbone of bisphosphonates.

Bisphosphonates differ from each other only at the two 'R' groups; R_1 is typically a hydroxyl group (–OH), whereas R_2 varies between bisphosphonates. This latter side chain determines the pharmacological properties of the drug. R_2 in the older drugs, such as clodronate, does not contain a nitrogen atom; these drugs behave differently to the newer agents, they work by inducing osteoclast apoptosis by generating a toxic analogue of adenosine triphosphate. Nitrogenous bisphosphonates, such as disodium pamidronate, ibandronic acid and zoledronic acid, act by binding and blocking the enzyme farnesyl diphosphate synthase (FPPS) in the HMG-CoA reductase pathway. FPPS is essential for normal osteoclast activity. It is noteworthy that statins also interfere with the HMG-CoA reductase pathway, but are not specific to bone. Research is currently underway to determine the effect of statins on bone metabolism.

7.2.2 Contraindications and precautions

- Avoid in pregnancy and breastfeeding
- Consider preventative dental work before starting bisphosphonate therapy due to the risk of osteonecrosis of the jaw
- Correct hypocalcaemia before initiating treatment
- Dose or rate of administration adjustments may be necessary in renal impairment
- Calcium supplements may be required.

7.2.3 Adverse effects

- Hypocalcaemia
- Hypomagnesaemia
- Hypophosphataemia
- Flu-like symptoms, including bone pain during infusion
- Nausea/vomiting
- Renal failure
- Osteonecrosis of the jaw.

Figure 7.1 Diagrammatic representation illustrating the similarity between pyrophosphate and bisphosphonates

Pyrophosphate

Basic structure of bisphosphonate

7.2.4 **Drug interactions**

Oral preparations should not be taken within at least 1 hour of calcium supplements, antacids or milk. Patients must drink adequate volumes of water to flush the drugs out of the oesophagus and should not lie down for an hour after taking the drug.

7.2.5 **Administration**

Doses for the treatment of bone pain are shown in Table 7.1.

Table 7.1 Doses of bisphosphonates for bone pain		
Drug	**Route**	**Dose**
Sodium clodronate	Oral	1.6 g daily in one or divided doses Must not be taken within at least 1 hour of food
	IV[*]	1500 mg in 500 ml sodium chloride 0.9% over at least 4 hours every 3–4 weeks
	SC[*]	1500 mg in 1000 ml sodium chloride 0.9% over 12–24 hours every 3–4 weeks (Walker et al., 1997)
Disodium pamidronate	IV	90 mg in 500 ml sodium chloride 0.9% at a rate not exceeding 1 mg/min
Ibandronic acid	IV	6 mg in 500 ml sodium chloride 0.9% over 1–2 hours every 3–4 weeks
	Oral	50 mg daily at least 1 hour before food or other medicine; patient must remain upright for at least 1 hour after taking
Zoledronic acid	IV	4 mg in 100 ml sodium chloride 0.9% over 15 minutes every 3–4 weeks. Patients should also be administered an oral calcium supplement of 500 mg and 400 IU vitamin D daily
[*] Unlicensed use.		

7.3 **Clonidine**

Clonidine is a mixed α_1 and α_2 adrenergic agonist, with the latter activity predominating. Generally encountered as an oral antihypertensive, clonidine can be administered via the epidural or intrathecal route for the treatment of pain. In addition, oral and transdermal clonidine administration can also be used for other poorly responsive pain. Transdermal clonidine patches are at present only available in the UK as unlicensed imports. Transdermal clonidine may possess both topical and systemic activity. Studies have shown analgesic benefits of clonidine in a variety of chronic pain conditions, including cancer, diabetic neuropathy and post herpetic neuralgia (Zeigler et al., 1992; Eisenach et al., 1995; Hassenbusch et al., 2002; Ackerman et al., 2003; Elkersh et al., 2003).

7.3.1 Pharmacology

The exact mechanism of action is unknown, but clonidine is thought to produce analgesia by directly acting on pre-synaptic and post-junctional α_2-adrenoceptors, thereby inhibiting pain transmission along adrenergic pathways within the spinal cord. Clonidine is metabolized to inactive metabolites and approximately 50% is excreted by the kidneys unchanged.

7.3.2 Contraindications and precautions

- Avoid in patients with severe bradyarrhythmia resulting from either sick sinus syndrome or AV block of second or third degree
- Avoid in pregnancy and breastfeeding; insufficient data are available
- Use with caution in patients with peripheral vascular disease, cerebrovascular or coronary insufficiency
- Do not withdraw abruptly due to risk of reactions e.g. rebound hypertension, agitation, anxiety and headache.

7.3.3 Adverse effects

The transdermal formulation is better tolerated than the oral route. The commonest adverse effects include:

- drowsiness
- hypotension
- dry mouth
- dizziness, presumably related to orthostatic hypotension.

7.3.4 Drug interactions

Drug interactions with clonidine are minimal and tend to be pharmacodynamic in nature, e.g. co-administration with an anti-hypertensive may increase the risk of hypotension. Combination with levomepromazine should be used cautiously since this can also precipitate orthostatic hypotension.

7.3.5 Administration

Clonidine is not licensed for the management of pain. It is available as a parenteral formulation that can be used intraspinally and as tablets for oral administration. A transdermal patch formulation can be obtained from outside the UK. Clonidine is reserved for use when more conventional treatments have failed. For systemic use, the dose is started low (e.g. 100 mcg po daily) and increased as necessary while monitoring for adverse effects such as hypotension that are dose-dependent. Intraspinally, clonidine is typically started at doses of

10–20 mcg/day, increasing up to a usual maximum of 150 mcg/day. Clonidine appears compatible with morphine, hydromorphone and bupivacaine (Classen *et al.*, 2004; Rudich *et al.*, 2004).

7.4 **Corticosteroids**

Corticosteroids (or steroids) have a multitude of clinical applications including treatment of pain. These drugs are often described as multipurpose analgesics and are widely used in the treatment of cancer pain syndromes (Mercadante *et al.*, 2001, 2007; Gannon & McNamara, 2002; Lundström & Fürst, 2006) including:

- bone pain
- headache from raised intracranial pressure
- neuropathic pain from nerve compression
- bowel obstruction.

In addition to the recognized benefit in conditions such as rheumatoid arthritis (Mellilo *et al.*, 2007), efficacy in other pain syndromes has been described, e.g. herpes zoster (but see 7.4.2) and chronic and chronic back pain (Santee, 2002; Abdi *et al.*, 2007).

7.4.1 **Pharmacology**

The pharmacological effects of steroids are diverse and are described in detail elsewhere (Rang *et al.*, 2007). The pharmacological mechanisms underlying the analgesic action remain unknown; several possibilities have been suggested:

- reduction in synthesis of peripheral inflammatory mediators, thereby reducing the excitation of nociceptors
- reduction of perineuronal and peritumoural oedema, reducing nerve compression
- direct inhibitory effect on hyperexcitable neurons.

Several steroids are available; in pain therapy dexamethasone, methylprednisolone and prednisolone are typically used. See Table 7.2 for equivalencies. Dexamethasone is often the agent of choice due to its relatively high potency and reduced mineralocorticoid effect. Steroids are well absorbed from the gastrointestinal tract and when applied topically. Metabolism occurs mainly in the liver and involves the cytochrome CYP3A4 system. Metabolites and any unchanged drug are excreted in the urine (Czock *et al.*, 2005).

7.4.2 **Contraindications and precautions**

- Avoid in patients with TB or chickenpox/shingles
- Avoid in patients with systemic illness, unless appropriate anti-infective agents are co-prescribed

- Avoid during pregnancy due to risk of cleft palate; breastfeeding probably safe with doses less than 40 mg prednisolone daily
- Withdrawal must be gradual after chronic therapy (see Box 7.1)
- Caution in patients with diabetes mellitus, congestive heart failure, hypertension, and previous or active peptic ulceration.

Table 7.2 Approximate equivalent anti-inflammatory doses of steroids

Steroid	Equivalent dose (mg)
Dexamethasone	7.5
Methylprednisolone	40
Prednisolone	50

Box 7.1 Steroid withdrawal

Abrupt cessation of steroid treatment is appropriate if:

- not more than 3 weeks treatment received
- disease state unlikely to relapse*
- not more than 40 mg prednisolone daily (or equivalent) received
- doses have not been taken at night (greater risk of adrenal cortical atrophy)
- no other cause(s) of adrenal insufficiency
- course not prescribed within 1 year of stopping long-term steroid therapy

* Steroids are not generally withdrawn abruptly in pain management. It is usual to decrease the dose gradually in order to either withdraw treatment or to determine a suitable maintenance dose, e.g.:

- dexamethasone 8–16 mg daily for 3–5 days
- reduce by 2 mg every 3–5 days until achieving maintenance dose or 2 mg daily
- to withdraw completely, reduce from 2 mg daily by 0.5 mg every 3–5 days

If steroid therapy has persisted beyond 3 weeks at doses greater than physiological (7.5 mg prednisolone or equivalent), then the dose can be rapidly reduced to physiological, providing relapse is unlikely. A slower reduction is then necessary before the steroid can be withdrawn. If relapse is likely, a more gradual dose reduction may be needed.

7.4.3 **Adverse Effects**

Table 7.3 lists examples of common steroid adverse effects.

Important
• Adverse effects are dose and duration dependent
• The chosen steroid will determine the extent of glucocorticoid and mineralocorticoid adverse effects
• Risk of peptic ulceration increases significantly if steroids are co-prescribed with a NSAID (including low-dose aspirin). Consider prophylaxis with a proton pump inhibitor or misoprostol.

Table 7.3 Steroid-induced adverse effects	
Adverse effect	**Notes**
Dyspepsia	Unless co-prescribed with NSAIDs and for short-term use only, a simple antacid should suffice. Ensure steroid taken with or after food
Hyperglycaemia	Ensure regular blood glucose monitoring or urine screening. Patient may require insulin therapy
Hypertension	Disruption of current anti-hypertensive treatment may occur
Immunosuppression	Patient must avoid contact with chickenpox or shingles if susceptible
Insomnia	Typically due to late afternoon, or evening dose. Ensure all doses are taken before 2 pm
Mental disturbances	May be related to peak plasma level. Increasing the frequency of doses may help. Some patients may require a continuous subcutaneous infusion, although this may increase the risk of insomnia and adrenal cortical atrophy

Other adverse effects include:

• weight gain
• myopathy
• osteoporosis (may require co-administration of bisphosphonate)
• hirsutism
• avascular osteonecrosis
• psychological manifestations.

7.4.4 **Drug interactions**

Pharmacokinetic interactions can occur with steroids given the hepatic metabolism by CYP3A4; drugs that affect the activity of this isozyme may interfere with steroid metabolism.

- Phenytoin—a complex interaction with dexamethasone as concentrations of both drugs can be affected; consider doubling the dose dexamethasone and monitoring plasma phenytoin concentrations
- Carbamazepine—consider doubling the dose of dexamethasone.

Pharmacodynamic interactions can occur with a variety of drugs given the wide ranging actions of steroids:

- NSAIDs—significant increase in risk of gastroduodenal toxicity; includes low-dose aspirin; ensure prophylactic gut protection prescribed
- Anti-hypertensives—reduced hypotensive effect due to steroid-induced sodium and water retention
- Digoxin—possible risk of increased toxicity, despite normal therapeutic digoxin ranges, due to steroid-induced hypokalaemia.

7.4.5 **Administration**

> **Important**
>
> - Use the lowest effective dose for the shortest time possible
> - Avoid doses after 2 pm; doses after this time may have a greater impact on adrenal cortical function and interfere with sleep
> - Ensure that the patient is reviewed and is not left on unnecessary long-term steroid therapy
> - Risks of prolonged steroid use, together with benefits, must be discussed with the patient.

The effective dose of steroid for the treatment of pain is unknown. The initial dose depends on the condition being treated. Dexamethasone is generally started at doses between 8 and 16 mg for cancer-related pain (although higher doses may be required if the patient is co-prescribed anti-epileptics). The dose is typically reduced after 3–5 days until the lowest effective dose is attained.

7.5 **Ketamine**

7.5.1 **Introduction**

Ketamine is a dissociative anaesthetic agent that was introduced over 40 years ago as a safer alternative to phencyclidine (PCP). Its popularity as an anaesthetic agent has declined because of the high incidence of disturbing emergence reactions, such as hallucinations and delirium that can persist for up to 24 hours. More recently, ketamine has been used in a variety of pain states at sub-anaesthetic doses, principally for conditions refractory to recognized therapy, e.g. peripheral and central neuropathic pain, ischaemic pain, cancer pain and breakthrough pain (Bell et al., 2003; Hocking & Cousins, 2003; Carr et al., 2004). Despite this, there are relatively few studies with adequate numbers of patients to easily determine the benefits and long-term effects of ketamine, or its place in chronic pain management.

7.5.2 Pharmacology

Ketamine has many central and peripheral pharmacological actions, including interaction with N-methyl-D-aspartate (NMDA) receptors, opioids receptors, muscarinic receptors and Na^+ ion channels (Hirota & Lambert, 1996). The analgesic effect of ketamine that is seen at sub-anaesthetic doses is due to non-competitive antagonism of the NMDA receptor (see Box 7.2). Ketamine interacts with the PCP binding site on the NMDA receptor (see Figure 7.2) blocking the influx of Na^+ and Ca^{2+}. Binding of ketamine only occurs when the ion channel has been opened though neuronal excitation. The analgesic activity is believed to be due to the attenuation of the 'wind-up' phenomenon by reducing the excitability of the neuron. Meaningful opioid effects may not occur until anaesthetic doses of ketamine are attained.

Ketamine is available commercially as a racemate, and the two stereoisomers, $S(+)$-ketamine and $R(-)$-ketamine, display different pharmacological properties. $S(+)$-ketamine appears to be a more potent antagonist of the NMDA receptor and is better tolerated than $R(-)$-ketamine. $S(+)$-ketamine is available in other countries and can be imported to the UK.

Box 7.2 The role of the NMDA receptor in chronic pain

The NMDA receptor is coupled to a non-specific ion channel. The receptor ion channel is blocked by Mg^{2+} in the resting state. Binding of phencyclidine (PCP) to the NMDA receptor at the aptly named PCP binding site also causes blockade of the ion channel. Activation of the NMDA receptor displaces Mg^{2+} resulting in the opening of the non-selective ion channel allowing Na^+ and Ca^{2+} to pass through thereby increasing the excitability of the neuron. In certain chronic pain conditions, continued C-fibre activation results in the hyperexcitability of spinal cord nociceptive neurons. This phenomenon of central sensitization is commonly referred to as 'wind-up.' The NMDA receptor is implicated in a variety of functions such as sensory perception (including persistent nociceptive and neuropathic pain), cognition and consciousness. It has been shown to have a major role in opioid tolerance and the development of chronic neuropathic pain.

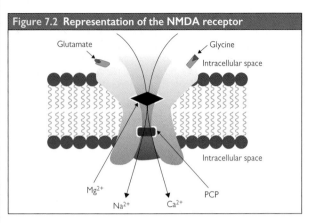

Figure 7.2 **Representation of the NMDA receptor**

Oral ketamine undergoes extensive first-pass hepatic metabolism to norketamine via the CYP3A4 cytochrome system. Although the analgesic potencies of ketamine and norketamine are thought to be the same, the peak plasma concentration of norketamine produced after oral administration is greater than that by parenteral. Consequently, the same analgesic effect appears to be achieved with lower oral doses compared with parenteral (Broadley *et al.*, 1996; Fitzgibbon *et al.*, 2002).

7.5.3 **Contraindications and precautions**

Ketamine must not be used in patients with:

- Severe coronary or myocardial disease
- Cerebrovascular accident
- Cerebral trauma
- Porphyria
- Avoid in pregnancy; after ketamine a newborn may be smaller than normal and have behavioural/learning problems
- Use with caution in patients at risk of raised intracranial pressure
- Use with caution in patients with a history of serious mental health problems.

7.5.4 **Adverse effects**

- Adverse effects are dose-dependent and psychotomimetic in nature
- Commencing ketamine at low doses and titrating slowly can reduce the incidence of adverse effects
- Converting from parenteral to oral administration allows for a dose reduction of up to 40%. This decreases the risk of adverse effects while the analgesic benefit is apparently maintained (Fitzgibbon *et al.*, 2002)

- Anxious patients may be more susceptible to these adverse effects, suggesting that the NMDA receptor ion channel is activated in this state. Co-administration of a benzodiazepine (e.g. diazepam 2 mg daily) or haloperidol (e.g. 1.5 mg daily) may reduce the incidence and severity of such effects (Hocking & Cousins, 2003; Villanueva-Perez et al., 2007)
- Psychotomimetic effects are less frequent in the young (<15 years) and the elderly (>65 years)
- Other less frequent adverse effects include increases in blood pressure, raised intracranial pressure, nausea and vomiting.
- Subcutaneous ketamine is irritant; site reactions have been reported during continuous subcutaneous infusion.

7.5.5 Drug interactions

Most clinically important drug interactions with ketamine are pharmacodynamic, e.g. increased sedation when midazolam and ketamine are co-administered. Given the importance of the cytochrome CYP3A4 in the metabolism of ketamine, caution should be used when co-administering drugs known to interfere with this enzyme, e.g. carbamazepine.

7.5.6 Administration

The dose of concurrent opioid should be reviewed as administration of ketamine can restore opioid sensitivity.

Ketamine is not currently licensed for the treatment of pain. A parenteral formulation, for general anaesthesia, is available and is utilized for subcutaneous use and the extemporaneous preparation of an oral formulation. An unlicensed oral solution is also available.

The dosing schedule for ketamine varies widely in the literature from low initial doses to high parenteral doses used for short duration (called burst ketamine therapy). Refer to Box 7.3 for a summary of ketamine dosage regimens.

Box 7.3 Dosing regimes for ketamine

Oral

Typically 50 mg/5 ml solution used
Usual starting dose 10 mg three to four times daily
Increase in steps of 20–40 mg/day
Max dose 100 mg four times daily; higher doses used with caution

CSCI

Usual starting dose 50–150 mg/day
Increase by 50–100 mg/day, to a max of 600 mg daily
Higher doses should be used with caution

Box 7.3 (Contd.)

Burst ketamine

Typically start at 100 mg/day via CSCI

Dose increased daily if no improvement by 100 mg

Typically given for 5 days, with max daily dose of 500 mg

Effect may persist for up to 2 months

Dose conversion

While no direct conversion exists, the oral analgesic dose is considered approximately **three times** more potent than the parenteral dose

7.5.7 Other analgesic drugs

Drugs that are less commonly encountered are shown in Table 7.4.

Table 7.4 Less commonly used analgesics			
Drug	**Indications**	**Dose**	**Notes**
Baclofen	Skeletal muscle relaxant (e.g. Motor Neurone Disease)	Oral: 5–10 mg twice or three times daily Max 100 mg/day	Adverse effects such as nausea and drowsiness can be minimized by using low initial doses Long-term treatment must not be suddenly withdrawn. Careful tapering is suggested
Calcitonin (Salmon)	Bone pain and neuro-pathic pain	SC: 100–200 IU once or twice daily	May cause nausea/vomiting which can be successfully treated with haloperidol. Subcutaneous test dose of 1 IU suggested in order to check for sensitivity
Nefopam	Chronic pain	Oral: 30–90 mg three times daily	Nefopam is chemically and pharmacologically distinct from any other analgesic. Its mode of action not fully understood but is believed to involve inhibition of monoamine re-uptake in the central nervous system. It has been shown to be opioid sparing and may have a role in neuropathic pain. Adverse effects include nausea, vomiting, hallucinations, dry mouth and urinary retention
Ziconotide	Severe chronic pain	Intrathecal, initially 2.4 mcg /day Max 21.6 mcg/day	Highly selective reversible blocker of N-type voltage-gated Ca^{2+} channels. Derived from venom of predatory sea snail, *conuz magus* Specialized use only

7.6 **Topical Analgesia**

7.6.1 **Introduction**

Injury within the periphery caused by chemical, mechanical or thermal stimuli triggers the release of several neuromodulators, such as adenosine triphosphate, protons (H^+) and prostaglandin E_2. Neuromodulators enable immediate detection of tissue damage through an excitatory effect on C and Aδ nociceptive fibres. In contrast, H^+ slowly accumulate after tissue damage and eventually cause pain (e.g. burning sensation) some time after the initial injury by activating the transient receptor potential V1 ion channel (TRPV1—see section 7.8). Prostaglandin E_2 production, although it occurs several hours after the initial injury, forms a major part of the inflammatory response. By binding to specific receptors on the cell membrane it changes the response of other receptors and ion channels, thereby indirectly increasing the excitability of the nociceptor. The effects of such action can be profound, e.g. after sunburn a warm shower becomes a painful experience because of prostaglandin-mediated increase in sensitivity of TRPV1 ion channels. In chronic inflammatory conditions, or after peripheral nerve injury, a nociceptive stimulus may not be necessary for signals to be transmitted, i.e. the pain outlasts the stimulus.

Topical analgesia provides an alternative option for the treatment of pain. Local application of a topical agent produces effects within the skin, soft tissue, and peripheral nerves without significant systemic absorption. This is in contrast to transdermal formulations that, although applied to the skin, require systemic absorption to be clinically active. Compared with systemic analgesics, topical agents possess several important advantages:

- low or negligible systemic absorption potentially negating the risk of adverse effects and drug interactions
- high local drug concentrations
- no dose titration
- ease of use.

The suitability, efficacy and tolerability of available topical preparations vary considerably. The benefits of topical analgesia in part depend on the degree of local inflammation, degree of peripheral nerve damage and the degree of central sensitization. The list of analgesics that can be applied topically is large and only commonly encountered treatments are discussed.

7.7 **Topical lidocaine 5% plaster**

Lidocaine is an amide local anaesthetic. Although its systemic use is discussed elsewhere (See Section 7.1), a topical formulation is also available. The hydrogel plaster (referred to as a plaster, rather than patch, to avoid confusion with transdermal analgesics) contains 700 mg of lidocaine (5% w/w) in an aqueous adhesive base. After 12 hours, 650 mg remains in the plaster and only 3% of the administered dose is absorbed systemically. In addition to the treatment of post-herpetic neuralgia, there is developing experience that suggests that topical lidocaine may be useful in other localized neuropathies (Argoff, 2006), osteoarthritis (Galer *et al.*, 2004) and low back pain (Argoff *et al.*, 2004).

7.7.1 Pharmacology

As with all local anaesthetics, lidocaine prevents the generation and conduction of nerve impulses by blocking sodium (Na^+) channels. As a general rule, small nerve fibres are more susceptible to the action of lidocaine than large fibres. Therefore, small diameter C and Aδ fibres, which mediate pain and temperature, are blocked before larger fibres that mediate, for example, touch and pressure. Lidocaine exhibits use-dependent block, i.e. it binds more tightly and rapidly to open channels and it appears to preferentially inhibit abnormal excessive activity at ectopic foci with increased Na^+ channel density. These conditions are present after peripheral nerve injury and in nociceptors sensitized by inflammatory modulators, e.g. prostaglandin E_2 (see above). The release characteristics of the lidocaine plaster are such that only very low concentrations penetrate the skin. Spontaneous ectopic discharges are suppressed by lidocaine applied topically and normal function is unaffected, i.e. the lidocaine plaster produces analgesia rather than anaesthesia.

7.7.2 Contraindications and precautions

- Avoid in patients with known hypersensitivity to amide anaesthetics
- Do not apply to inflamed or broken skin
- Manufacturer advises caution in patients with severe cardiac, renal or hepatic impairment.

7.7.3 Adverse effects

Adverse effects are generally localized reactions, commonly being administration site reactions such as erythema, rash, site irritation and pruritus. Appropriate use of the plaster is unlikely to cause systemic adverse reactions because the systemic absorption of lidocaine is very low.

7.7.4 Administration

The lidocaine plaster is currently indicated for the treatment of neuropathic pain associated with post-herpetic neuralgia. Up to three plasters can be applied to unbroken skin for 12 hours within a 24-hour period, with a subsequent plaster-free interval of at least 12 hours. The plasters can be cut to size. There may be a response within an hour of applying the plaster, although this may be due to the hydrogel formulation, rather than the active ingredient. Patients should be given an adequate trial of up to 4 weeks therapy before discontinuing treatment. Used plasters should be disposed of by folding the adhesive layers so that they stick together; the plaster will still contain active ingredient so due care is advised.

7.8 Topical capsaicin

Capsaicin is the constituent of chilli peppers that gives them the characteristic 'hot' taste. Topical capsaicin has been used for a variety of localized neuropathies. A recent systematic review concluded that topical capsaicin has moderate to poor efficacy in the treatment of chronic musculoskeletal or neuropathic pain (Mason *et al.*, 2004). Topical capsaicin is generally not a satisfactory sole treatment option for chronic pain conditions and it is often considered an adjuvant after other approaches have failed.

7.8.1 Pharmacology

The precise mechanism of action of capsaicin is currently unknown, although it is believed to involve TRPV1 ion channel, substance P and a proposed reversible direct neurotoxic effect. The TRPV1 ion channel is present on both C and Aδ fibres and activation by capsaicin and its analogues, heat, acidification, and lipid metabolites produces a characteristic burning sensation. Upon application, capsaicin initially produces nociceptor excitation through activation of TRPV1 ion channels and release of neurotransmitters, including substance P. Continued application of capsaicin produces analgesia through reversible desensitization (which may involve tachyphylaxis and a degree of loss of sensory fibres) (Nolano *et al.*, 1999).

7.8.2 Contraindications and precautions

- Must not be used on broken or inflamed skin
- Keep away from eyes and mucous membranes
- Wash hands immediately after application.

7.8.3 Adverse effects

The most frequently reported adverse effect with capsaicin is burning at the site of application that can lead to reduced patient compliance and treatment failure. Unless it is applied frequently and regularly for at least 4 weeks it will not be effective and this leads to problems with compliance. The burning sensation is more likely to occur if capsaicin is applied less frequently than 3–4 times daily, or just before or after a shower or bath. Patients should be reminded to wash their hands thoroughly after application to prevent contamination.

7.8.4 **Administration**

Capsaicin is currently available as a cream, in two strengths: 0.025% and 0.075%. The former is licensed for the symptomatic relief of pain associated with osteoarthritis while the latter is licensed for the symptomatic relief of post-herpetic neuralgia and painful diabetic peripheral neuropathy. A small amount of capsaicin cream should be applied to affected area 3–4 times a day. The application area must be unbroken. A trial of at least 4 weeks is necessary before reviewing treatment. If successful, the application can be slowly reduced to twice daily.

7.9 **Nonsteroidal anti-inflammatory drugs (NSAIDs)**

NSAIDs are the most widely prescribed drugs worldwide and have a pivotal role in the management of chronic pain. Topical NSAIDs are available in a variety of proprietary formulations, including gels and a medicated plaster. The efficacy of topical NSAIDs has been controversial, with the belief that any analgesic benefit is due to systemic absorption or a high incidence of placebo effect. However, a systematic review and meta-analysis concluded that topical NSAIDs were effective and safe in treating chronic musculoskeletal conditions (Mason et al., 2004).

7.9.1 **Pharmacology**

The pharmacology of the NSAIDs is discussed in Section 2.2. Although undoubtedly useful analgesics, NSAIDs carry a risk of clinically significant adverse effects, ranging from troublesome dyspepsia to peptic ulceration, bleeding, renal failure and myocardial infarction. Apart from the development of less toxic systemic drugs based on NSAID pharmacology, such as licofelone (Alvaro-Gracia, 2004) or naproxcinod (Ongini and Bolla, 2006), an alternative approach to reduce the risk of adverse effects is the use of topical therapy. Prostaglandin E_2 is implicated in peripheral sensitization, but these drugs will have no effect on immediate nociceptive inflammatory pain because prostanoid production is delayed until several hours after initial injury. Systemic absorption of topical NSAIDs is minimal, with plasma concentrations ranging from 5–15% of those achieved by systemic therapy. After topical application, local concentration of NSAID is relatively high in the dermal layer, but concentrations in tissue below the application site are similar to those attained through systemic therapy (Heyneman et al., 2000). Whether this is due to local penetration or systemic absorption, remains unclear. Nonetheless, topical NSAIDs represent a safe and effective treatment option.

7.9.2 Contraindications and precautions

- Avoid in the third trimester of pregnancy
- Do not apply to broken or inflamed skin
- Systemic absorption does occur but is unlikely to produce systemic adverse effects.

7.9.3 Adverse effects

Topical NSAIDs are generally well-tolerated. Mild local effects may occur in 10–15% of patients, e.g. erythema, pruritus or dermatitis. Topical NSAIDs rarely induce systemic adverse effects, although dyspepsia and nausea have been reported.

7.9.4 Administration

Gel formulations of NSAIDs are typically applied 3–4 times daily to unbroken skin.

7.10 Topical opioids

Although there are no commercially available topical opioid formulations, the administration of opioids by this route has been well documented. Typically, morphine sulphate or diamorphine hydrochloride are used, having been mixed in a vehicle such as Intrasite® gel. Several studies have reported that opioids applied topically to painful ulcers or lesions have analgesic properties (Twillman et al., 1999; Zeppetella et al., 2003).

7.10.1 Pharmacology

Three opioid receptors, μ, δ and κ, have been identified on the peripheral terminals of C and Aδ fibres; they are not usually prominent pharmacological targets until after inflammatory changes occur. Activation of peripheral opioid receptors results in attenuation of the excitability of nerve terminals with resultant analgesia. In contrast to other topical analgesics, opioids have to be applied to inflamed, often broken skin to be effective.

7.10.2 Adverse effects

The incidence of adverse effects with topical opioids, e.g. morphine or diamorphine appears to be minimal, as systemic absorption is negligible in most cases. However, as the application area increases in size, so does the risk of systemic absorption.

7.10.3 Administration

A commercial preparation is unavailable. Prescriptions will require extemporaneous preparation. A concentration of 1 mg/ml (0.1% w/v) is often used initially, although higher concentrations may be necessary (e.g. up to 0.5% w/v). The amount of gel to apply depends on the application area; usually up to 10 ml is applied—two to three times daily. A dressing, such as a vapour permeable film, is used to cover the wound. Combination of diamorphine or morphine with Intrasite® gel has been shown to be chemically stable for up to 28 days (Zeppetella et al., 2005). However, these formulations are not sterile and should be applied once prepared.

7.10.4 Miscellaneous

A variety of adjuvant drugs have been applied topically, but these should not be used in preference to a recognized more evidence-based treatment. Doxepin is available as a 5% cream and is indicated for the treatment of pruritus. It has been used successfully to treat neuropathic pain (McCleane, 2000). Doxepin mouthwash has been used to effectively treat oral mucositis, a common and painful condition that affects cancer patients (Epstein et al., 2007). The exact mechanism of action of doxepin as a peripheral analgesic is unknown.

The discovery of glutamate receptors on unmyelinated nerves in the skin that are upregulated after inflammation or nerve injury possibly prompted the use of topical ketamine. The mechanism of action of ketamine remains unclear, but it may involve interaction with Na^+ channels and peripheral opioid receptors. Ketamine is not available commercially in a topical formulation and its systemic use is discussed in Section 7.5. Nonetheless, there are several case reports of successful use of extemporaneously prepared topical ketamine (Gammaitoni et al., 2000; Slatkin and Rhiner, 2003).

Other drugs have been applied topically in extemporaneous formulations, with anecdotal reports of success. At present, the topical use of drugs such as clonidine and gabapentin should only be used in patients unable to tolerate conventional treatments.

Key references

Abdi S, Datta S, Trescot AM, et al. (2007). Epidural steroids in the management of chronic spinal pain: a systematic review. Pain Physician 10: 85–212.

Ackerman LL, Follett KA, Rosenquist RW (2003). Long-term outcomes during treatment of chronic pain with intrathecal clonidine or clonidine/opioid combinations. J. Pain Symptom Manage. 26: 668–77.

Alvaro-Gracia JM (2004). Licofelone—clinical update on a novel LOX/COX inhibitor for the treatment of osteoarthritis. Rheumatology 43 (Suppl 1): i21–5.

Argoff CE (2006). Topical agents for the treatment of chronic pain. Curr. Pain Headache Rep. 10: 11–19.

Argoff CE, Galer BS, Jensen MP, et al. (2004). Effectiveness of the lidocaine patch 5% on pain qualities in three chronic pain states: assessment with the Neuropathic Pain Scale. Curr. Med. Res. Opin. 20 (Suppl 2): S21–8.

Bell R, Eccleston C, Kalso E (2003). Ketamine as an adjuvant to opioids for cancer pain. *Cochr. Database Syst. Rev.* **1**: CD003351.

Broadley KE, Kurowska A, Tookman A (1996). Ketamine injection used orally. *Palliat. Med.* **10**: 247–50.

Bruera E, Ripamonti C, Brennis C, et al. (1992). A randomized double-blind controlled trial of intravenous lidocaine in the treatment of neuropathic cancer patients. *J. Pain Symptom Manage.* **7**: 138–40.

Carr DB, Goudas LC, Denman WT, et al. (2004). Safety and efficacy of intranasal ketamine for the treatment of breakthrough pain in patients with chronic pain: a randomized, double-blind, placebo-controlled, crossover study. *Pain* **108**: 17–27.

Challapalli V, Tremont-Lukats IW, McNicol ED, et al. (2005). Systemic administration of local anesthetic agents to relieve neuropathic pain. *Cochr. Database Syst. Rev.* **4**: CD003345.

Classen AM, Wimbish GH, Kupiec TC (2004). Stability of admixture containing morphine sulfate, bupivacaine hydrochloride, and clonidine hydrochloride in an implantable infusion system. *J. Pain Symptom Manage.* **28**: 603–11.

Cralow J, Tripathy D (2007). Managing metastatic bone pain: the role of bisphosphonates. *J. Pain Symptom Manage.* **33**: 462–72.

Czock D, Keller F, Rasche FM, Haussler U (2005). Pharmacokinetics and pharmacodynamics of systemically administered glucocorticoids. *Clin. Pharmacokinet.* **44**: 61–98.

Eisenach JC, DuPen S, Dubois M, et al. (1995). Epidural clonidine analgesia for intractable cancer pain. The Epidural Clonidine Study Group. *Pain* **61**: 391–9.

Eisenberg E, Geller R, Ball S (2007). Pharmacotherapy options for complex regional pain syndrome. *Expert. Rev. Neurother.* **7**: 521–31.

Ellemann K, Sjogren P, Banning AM, et al. (1989). Trial of intravenous lidocaine on painful neuropathy in cancer patients. *Clin. J. Pain* **5**: 291–4.

Elkersh MA, Simopoulos TT, Malik AB, et al. (2003). Epidural clonidine relieves intractable neuropathic itch associated with herpes zoster-related pain. *Reg. Anesth. Pain Med.* **28**: 344–6.

Epstein JB, Epstein JD, Epstein MS, et al. (2007). Management of pain in cancer patients with oral mucositis: follow-up of multiple doses of doxepin oral rinse. *J. Pain Symptom Manage.* **33**: 111–14.

Fitzgibbon EJ, Hall P, Schroder C, et al. (2002). Low dose ketamine as an analgesic adjuvant in difficult pain syndromes: a strategy for conversion from parenteral to oral ketamine. *J. Pain Symptom Manage.* **23**: 165–70.

Galer BS, Sheldon E, Patel N, et al. (2004). Topical lidocaine patch 5% may target a novel underlying pain mechanism in osteoarthritis. *Curr. Med. Res. Opin.* **20**: 1455–8.

Gammaitoni A, Gallagher RM, Walz-Bosna M (2000). Topical ketamine gel: possible role in treating neuropathic pain. *Pain Med.* **1**: 97–100.

Gannon C, McNamara P (2002). A retrospective observation of corticosteroid use at the end of life in a hospice. *J. Pain Symptom Manage.* **24**: 328–34.

Hasking D (2006). Pharmacological therapy of Paget's and other metabolic bone diseases. *Bone* **38** (Suppl 2): S3–7.

Hassenbusch SJ, Gunes S, Wachsman S, Willis KD (2002). Intrathecal clonidine in the treatment of intractable pain: a phase I/II study. *Pain Med.* **3**: 85–91.

Heyneman CA, Lawless-Liday C, Wall GC (2000). Oral versus topical NSAIDs in rheumatic diseases. A comparison. *Drugs* **60**: 555–74.

Hirota K, Lambert DG (1996). Ketamine: its mechanism(s) of action and unusual clinical uses. *Br. J. Anaesth.* **77**: 441–4.

Hocking G, Cousins MJ (2003). Ketamine in chronic pain management: an evidence-based review. *Anesth. Analg.* **9**: 1730–9.

Lundström SH, Fürst CJ (2006). The use of corticosteroids in Swedish palliative care. *Acta. Oncol.* **45**: 430–7.

Mason L, Moore RA, Derry S, et al. (2004). Systematic review of topical capsaicin for the treatment of chronic pain. *Br. Med. J.* **328**: 991–5.

Mason L, Moore RA, Edwards JE, et al. (2004). Topical NSAIDs for chronic musculoskeletal pain: systematic review and meta-analysis. *BMC Musculoskel. Disord.* **5**: 28.

McCleane G (2000). Topical doxepin hydrochloride reduces neuropathic pain: a randomized, double-blind, placebo-controlled study. *Pain Clinic* **12**: 47–50.

Mellilo N, Corrado A, Quarta L, Cantatore FP (2007). Corticosteroids, a review. *Panminerva Med.* **49**: 29–33.

Mercadante S, Casuccio A, Mangione S (2007). Medical treatment of inoperable malignant bowel obstruction. *J. Pain Symptom Manage.* **33**: 217–23.

Mercadante S, Fulfaro F, Casuccio A (2001). The use of corticosteroids in home palliative care. *Support. Cancer Care* **9**: 386–9.

Nolano M, Simone DA, Wendelschafer-Crabb G, et al. (1999). Topical capsaicin in humans: parallel loss of epidermal nerve fibres and pain sensation. *Pain* **81**: 135–45.

Ongini E, Bolla M (2006). Nitric oxide based nonsteroidal anti-inflammatory agents. *Drug Discov. Today Ther. Strateg.* **3**: 395–400.

Rang HP, Dale MM, Ritter JM, Flower R (2007). *Rang and Dale's Pharmacology*, 6th edn. Churchill Livingstone, Oxford.

Rudich Z, Peng P, Dunn E, McCartney C (2004). Stability of clonidine in clonidine-hydromorphone mixture from implanted intrathecal infusion pumps in chronic pain patients. *J. Pain Symptom Manage.* **28**: 599–602.

Santee JA (2002). Corticosteroids for herpes zoster. What do they accomplish? *Am. J. Clin. Dermatol.* **3**: 517–24.

Slatkin NE, Rhiner M (2003). Topical ketamine in the treatment of mucositis pain. *Pain Med.* **4**: 298–303.

Sloan P, Basta M, Storey P, von Gunten C (1999). Mexiletine as an adjuvant analgesic for the management of neuropathic cancer pain. *Anesth. Analg.* **89**: 760–1.

Tremont-Lukats IW, Hutson PR, Backonja MM (2006). A randomized, double-masked, placebo-controlled pilot trial of extended IV lidocaine infusion for relief of ongoing neuropathic pain. *Clin. J. Pain* **22**: 266–71.

Twillman RK, Long TD, Cathers TA, Mueller DW (1999). Treatment of painful skin ulcers with topical opioids. *J. Pain Symptom Manage.* **17**: 288–92.

Villanueva-Perez VL, Cerda-Olmedo G, Samper JM, *et al.* (2007). Oral ketamine for the treatment of type I complex regional pain syndrome. *Pain Pract.* **7**: 39–43.

Walker P, Watanabe S, Lawlor P, *et al.* (1997). Subcutaneous clodronate: a study evaluating efficacy in hypercalcemia of malignancy and local toxicity. *Ann. Oncol.* **8**: 915–16.

Wong R, Wiffen PJ (2002). Bisphosphonates for the relief of pain secondary to bone metastases. *Cochr. Database Syst. Rev.* **2**: CD002068.

Yuen KK, Shelley M, Sze WM, Wilt T, Mason MD (2006). Bisphosphonates for advanced prostate cancer. *Cochr. Database Syst. Rev.* **4**: CD006250.

Zeigler D, Lynch SA, Muir J, *et al.* (1992). Transdermal clonidine versus placebo in painful diabetic neuropathy. *Pain* **48**: 403–8.

Zeppetella G, Joel S, Ribeiro M (2005). Stability of morphine sulphate and diamorphine hydrochloride in intrasite gel. *Palliat. Med.* **19**: 131–6.

Zeppetella G, Paul J, Ribeiro MDC (2003). Analgesic efficacy of morphine applied topically to painful ulcers. *J. Pain Symptom Manage.* **25**: 555–8.

Chapter 8

Interventional techniques for chronic pain

Brigitta Brandner and M. Nagaratnam

> **Key points**
>
> - Interventional anaesthetic techniques provide clinicians with a useful tool for the diagnosis and treatment of chronic pain
> - Techniques used include intravenous techniques, peripheral and central nerve blocks, and autonomic blocks.
> - The main contraindications to the use of interventional techniques are related to the patient's psychological state or medical condition
> - There must be rapid and clear communication with primary care teams about aftercare following interventions.

8.1 Introduction

Interventional anaesthetic techniques have been a mainstay of pain treatment for many years and still have a firm place in its management. The principle is to modulate pain along its pathway from peripheral to central transmission. The clinician has to have a sound knowledge of the origin of the pain including its anatomy and pathophysiology. Interventions must be performed in a multidisciplinary team structure with support from a variety of health care professionals.

8.2 Principles

Intravenous techniques, peripheral and central nerve blocks and autonomic blocks are possible.

8.2.1 General

- A detailed and complete history has to be obtained with emphasis on the indications for any intervention

- The main contraindications are local (e.g. infection) or related to the patient's psychological state (e.g. unwillingness or inability to understand and/or consent to the procedure) or medical condition (e.g. frailty, coagulopathy, immune suppression and impending spinal cord compression) or no provision for aftercare
- As for any operative procedure the patient should be appropriately prepared, e.g. fasted, any medical co-morbidity optimized and they must not be allergic to the medications to be used
- Informed consent has to be sought before the procedure with a detailed explanation of risks and benefits and enough time to consider the options
- The procedures have to be performed in a safe clinical environment where sterility can be maintained, assistance by trained staff, with fluoroscopy or CT scanner available as required, and resuscitation equipment to hand
- Basic monitoring standards apply
- Aseptic techniques have to be followed for all interventions
- After the procedure, the patient must recover in designated areas supervised by trained staff
- Patients must be discharged with a treatment plan for managing complications, e.g. what to do about a pneumothorax
- There must be rapid and clear communication with primary care teams about aftercare following all interventions.

8.2.2 Sedation

Depending on the nature of the procedure or patient, sedation should be administered by an independent operator. Short-acting drugs such as midazolam, remifentanil, alfentanil and propofol are preferred. Sedation must be minimal when implanting spinal or peripheral nerve stimulation electrodes so that the patient can communicate with the operator about the effects of stimulation.

8.2.3 Nerve stimulators

For specific nerve blocks a nerve stimulator is required. Mixed nerves can be isolated by stimulating motor function without eliciting pain by limiting current intensity and duration (0.05–0.2 ms), longer pulse durations (0.3–1.0 ms) test sensory supply. Applying current via the cathode (negative electrode adjacent to nerve) significantly reduces current required for response. Nerve stimulation needles can vary but an insulated bevelled needle improves the accuracy by confining the current to the tip.

8.2.4 Solutions used for nerve blocking

Blocks conducted for the management of chronic pain may produce transient effects as with local anaesthetic, mid-range as with depot steroids or be more permanent as with neurolytic drugs, e.g. phenol.

Transient blocks are conducted with local anaesthetic for diagnostic and therapeutic purposes. The local anaesthetic most commonly used is lidocaine 1% with maximum dose calculated per body weight of 3 mg/kg. Bupivacaine has been used but it is cardiotoxic in doses of more than 2 mg/kg. Levo-bupivacaine has the advantage of being less cardiotoxic at the same dose and it should be the agent of choice when a longer action is needed.

A depot steroid is sometimes added to the injectate; it is diluted with 10–15 mL of local anaesthetic. The steroid preparation most commonly used is methylprednisolone acetate or triamcinolone diacetate. A possible mechanism of steroid action reflects inhibition of phospholipase A2 resulting in decreased synthesis of prostaglandins. However, there are numerous other putative mechanisms, e.g. alteration of local blood flow and nerve growth factors.

Neurolysis is the long-lasting or permanent interruption of neural transmission, as a result of therapeutic application of a chemical or physical destructive agent to a nerve. It is used only after the effectiveness of the nerve block has been established usually by a test dose of simple local anaesthetic. The drugs used in neurolysis are chemical neurolytic agents; alcohol (concentration of at least 50% are needed; probably 75% for coeliac block) or phenol (commonly as a 6% solution). The use of neurolytic on peripheral nerves may lead to deafferentation pain after the nerves regenerate and must therefore be used selectively. Neurolysis may also be performed with cold (cryotherapy) and heat (radiofrequency lesioning).

8.2.5 Fluoroscopy, CT scan and ultrasound

For fluoroscopy usually a C arm is required, as both lateral and AP views are necessary to ensure correct needle placement. The operator should be appropriately trained. Repeated procedures can lead to increasing radiation exposure. Gun barrel technique is commonly used (needle placement parallel to X-ray beam). CT guidance confers better target visualization at the expense of significantly higher radiation exposure. Radio-opaque contrast is commonly used to identify the anatomic structures under fluoroscopy or CT guidance. For central blockade, water-soluble non-ionic agents such as metrizamide are needed.

Many joint injections are more accurate when ultrasound guidance is used (Eichenberger U et al., 2004). Ultrasound guidance is also proving to be feasible for peripheral nerve blocks; direct visualization of the nerve improves accuracy, reducing volume of drug with no radiation involved. However, sound anatomical knowledge and technical skill in handling a transducer in combination with a needle are required.

8.3 **Intravenous techniques**

8.3.1 **Intravenous drug challenges**

When oral therapy is ineffective or side effects are intolerable then intravenous routes are sometimes preferred. Rapid onset and reliable pharmacokinetics are needed to assess the effectiveness of the agent chosen. The duration of the analgesic effect can outlive the plasma half-life of the drug; this may be due to neural remodelling. Intravenous drug challenges can aid in the diagnosis of the underlying pathophysiological process of neuropathic and/or sympathetically maintained pains. However, great care is needed to allow for the predictable placebo response to intravenous drug administration.

Lidocaine

Intravenous (IV) infusions of local anaesthetic have been known for over 50 years to alleviate pain in a wide variety of conditions including neuropathies. The pain relieving effect can be of significantly greater duration than the half-life of the drug. Some patients experience weeks of pain relief following an infusion. Lidocaine is a suitable local anaesthetic as its potential cardiovascular side effects are uncommon in the doses used for the infusion.

Ketamine

Ketamine acts at a number of receptors, but principally as an N-methyl-D-aspartate (NMDA) antagonist. NMDA receptors are sited peripherally and centrally. Activation of the receptor results in the development of hyperalgesia and allodynia. Ketamine is used clinically in chronic pain states such as complex regional pain syndrome (CRPS), fibromyalgia, ischaemic and neuropathic pain. Sub-anaesthetic doses reduce temporal summation and can decrease requirement for analgesic medication. Side effects such as nightmares, hallucinations and psychomimetic effects can limit its use long term. Intravenous test doses of ketamine may not predict the effects of oral ketamine that probably acts as a pro-drug for nor-ketamine. It is also sometimes difficult to organize for this drug to be prescribed in a primary care setting.

Opioids

An intravenous opioid challenge can be useful in assessing the reduction/response of pain to opioids before initiating long-term oral opioid therapy. A short-acting opioid is used such as fentanyl, alfentanil and remifentanil. Respiratory depression and nausea can be a problem. A single response does not always predict long-term opioid efficacy.

Phentolamine

Sympathetic blockade can be achieved by pharmacological manipulation of the α1-adrenergic receptor by an antagonist. Phentolamine is a reversible non-selective α-adrenergic antagonist whose primary action is vasodilation. It can have a diagnostic role in CRPS. It can be infused (0.5 mg/kg) in the outpatient setting as a diagnostic tool for some neuropathic pains. Patients should be pre-treated with intravenous fluids followed by propranolol and fully monitored. A good response may indicate sympathetically maintained pain.

Phenytoin sodium

Phenytoin sodium is a commonly used anti-epileptic drug that inhibits seizures by stabilizing the inactive state of voltage-gated sodium channels. Phenytoin was the first oral antiepileptic to be used as an analgesic in neuropathic pain. It may be effective in reducing burning and shooting pain, sensitivity, numbness, when given as an infusion of 15 mg/kg over 2 hours. The pain relief may outlast both the infusion time and plasma half-life of phenytoin. This may be used to treat flare-ups of some chronic neuropathic pain.

8.3.2 Intravenous regional sympathetic blockade

Sympathetic modulation with drugs such as guanethidine, bretylium or local anaesthetic given peripherally has been a traditional approach to diagnosing and treating CRPS. Guanethidine acts by temporarily displacing norepinephrine from adrenergic nerve endings. A tourniquet is applied to the affected extremity and inflated. A predetermined dose of the drug is injected into the isolated limb and the tourniquet is released after appropriate time (usually 20 minutes). Often a series of blocks is performed to assess the response. There is insufficient evidence of the long-term benefit of this treatment in isolation; trials of its combination with exercise and rehabilitation are lacking.

8.4 Local anaesthetic injections

8.4.1 Myofascial trigger point injections

Myofascial trigger points (MTPs) need to be differentiated from simple generalized tender points. Every muscle has a potential trigger point that can become painful. Trigger points are discrete, focal, hyperirritable spots located in a taut band of skeletal muscle. They trigger pain from the source point to the satellite point. MTPs often accompany chronic musculoskeletal disorders. It is necessary to distinguish between myofascial pain and nerve root pain (Alvarez & Rockwell 2002). Myofascial pain is due solely to activation of trigger points. Acute trauma or repetitive microtrauma may stress muscle fibres and lead to the formation of trigger points. Specific treatment of MTPs is aimed at reducing local and referred pain by injecting local anaesthetic or other agents, e.g. depot steroid or botulinium toxin.

8.4.2 Indications (Table 8.1)

Table 8.1 Indications for MTP injections	
MTPs	**Tender points**
Local tenderness, taut band, local twitch response, jump sign	Local tenderness
Single or multiple	Multiple
May occur in any skeletal muscle	Occur in specific locations that are often symmetrically located
May cause a specific referred pain pattern	Do not cause referred pain, but often cause a total body pain sensitivity
Not associated with systemic manifestations	Often associated with systemic manifestations of a fibromyalgia type, e.g. sleep disturbance

MTPs and not tender points should be treated and these can be differentiated using the above criteria.

8.4.3 **Contraindications**
- Uncorrectable anticoagulation or bleeding disorders
- Caution with aspirin and clopidogrel
- Local or systemic infection
- Allergy to agents to be injected
- Acute muscle trauma.

8.4.4 **Technique**
The patient should be placed in a comfortable or recumbent position to produce muscle relaxation. Sedation is not required.
- Flat palpation to locate MTP
- Needle insertion 1–2 cm away from MTP
- Advance slowly painful area
- End point—a sharp pain and muscle twitching as needle connects with the muscular taut band
- Negative aspiration to detect intravascular needling
- Inject solution slowly
- Withdraw needle to the level of the subcutaneous tissue
- Redirect superiorly, inferiorly, laterally and medially, repeating the needling and injection process in each direction until the local twitch response is no longer elicited
- Gentle muscle stretching is often useful immediately after the injection and then on a regular basis.

8.4.5 **Special points**
Steroids can be added to the injectate solution; however, this can lead to fat and muscle necrosis especially if repeated. Botulinium toxin may be used. This takes 2 weeks to have an effect that lasts about 4 months.

8.4.6 **Side effects**

- Vasovagal syncope
- Immediate post-injection soreness that can persist for 3–4 days
- Skin infection
- Needle breakage; avoid by never inserting the needle to its hub
- Haematoma.

8.4.7 **Benefits and repeatability**

- Repeated injections in a particular muscle are not recommended if two or three previous attempts have been unsuccessful
- Patients should be encouraged to remain active but avoid strenuous activity, especially in the first 3–4 days after injection.

8.5 **Sympathetic blocks**

These may involve the cervical, thoracic and lumbar sympathetic chains. In theory, sympathetically mediated or maintained pain can be modulated by interrupting the transmission of pain in the nervous system. The use of neural sympathetic blockade for diagnostic, therapeutic, prognostic and treatment of chronic pain is well established. The evidence base is often quite weak, but individual clinicians often report anecdotally good results in some refractory cases.

8.5.1 **Indications**

- Sympathetic blockade can be useful in CRPS and sympathetically mediated pain
- There is evidence for effectiveness in ischaemic conditions such as peripheral vascular disease and diabetes (particularly with the involvement of small vessels and rest pain), Raynauds and refractory angina pectoris
- Visceral pain arising from the renal tract or pancreas can respond well
- Pain from a variety of gastrointestinal or pelvic malignancies may be helped
- In severe cases of hyperhydrosis, sympathectomy can be useful
- Bilateral sympathectomy may help with malignant tenesmus.

8.5.2 **Contraindications**

- Ischaemic pain due occlusion of larger vessels (claudication) or venous insufficiency, when further investigation is often necessary
- Uncorrectable coagulopathy
- Recent myocardial infarction or cardiac arrhythmia
- Glaucoma
- Anatomical problems in some cases, e.g. aortic aneurysm may make lumbar sympathectomy difficult or malignancy may lead to large nodes that hamper coeliac plexus block.

8.5.3 **Common complications and side effects with all sympathetic blocks**

- Haematoma
- Allergic reaction
- Central side effects of local anaesthetic
- Infection
- Each block also has some more specific risks (see below).

8.6 **Stellate ganglion block**

8.6.1 **Techniques**

The patient is positioned supine, sitting up at 45°, head extended, arms down by the sides. The mouth should be held open to slacken the strap muscles. The patient must not speak during the block as this moves the landmarks. Traditionally, this block is performed using anatomical landmarks however radiological screening can be used. The cricoid cartilage is located at the level of C6, with the carotid artery laterally. A remote needle technique is preferable with two operators. A 25 G needle is inserted perpendicular to the skin until the transverse process of C6 (Chaissaignac's tubercle) is located; the needle is then withdrawn minimally. A solution of 10–20 mL of 1% lidocaine is injected slowly after negative aspiration with assessment of any central or cardiac side effects. Other local anaesthetics or agents such as bupivacaine, levobupivicaine, morphine or buprenorphine have been used with limited evidence. Techniques using X-ray, CT scan and ultrasound guidance are evolving; it has been suggested that less solution is adequate to achieve a good result (Erickson & Hogan 1993). The patient is positioned supine, head extended, arms down by the side. In the lateral view the C7 vertebral body is located and a 25 G needle directed medially, caudally and posterior to hit transverse process and rolled of slightly. An AP view is then taken to confirm the correct needle position before injection of the therapeutic agent.

8.6.2 **End points**

Horner's syndrome (ipsilateral meiosis, ptosis, enophthalmos and nasal congestion) is an almost invariable sign of a successful block of the face; it does not guarantee that the arm is blocked. An increase in temperature in the affected extremity of at least 3°C from the baseline is more specific in detecting a successful block of the arm. Temperatures are measured by hand thermistors on the patient's middle digits.

8.6.3 **Complications and side effects**

The block should only be performed unilaterally as phrenic nerve palsy and pneumothorax are rare complications. Intravascular injection with local anaesthetic and central effects can be serious complications as are cardiac arrhythmias. Recurrent laryngeal nerve paralysis is characterized by a hoarse voice and swallowing problems.

8.6.4 Benefits and repeatability

For angina management, this block can be repeated many times; repeated blocks are required for its continued efficacy. There is evidence in animal models that the optimal lidocaine concentration is 1%.

8.7 Thoracic sympathectomy

Endoscopic thoracic sympathectomy is performed by surgeons and requires a general anaesthetic. Access is via the pectoral folds in the armpit by passing a fibre optic scope; this is similar to performing a thoracoscopy. Immediate risks are mainly due to one-lung anaesthesia. This procedure can cure almost 90% of upper limb hyperhydrosis. A specific side effect is the occurrence of compensatory sweating elsewhere; this cannot be predicted and can be irreversible and highly disturbing.

8.8 Lumbar sympathetic block

8.8.1 Technique

This can be done with the patient prone with a pillow under abdomen and the arms forward under the head or in the lateral position. The procedure is always performed under X-ray guidance; the use of ultrasound has been described. The body of lumbar vertebrae L3 is located (counting from T12 with the rib visible). The needle entry is usually 7–8 cm on either side from midline (spinous process). A 20G 20-cm needle is aimed anteriorly, medially and cranially hitting the bony L3 vertebral body (checked in two planes). It is then slid forwards so it comes to rest posterior to the anterior vertebral body through the psoas sheath (often a 'click' is felt). Contrast material is injected to ensure good spread that is parallel to the vertebral bodies and to exclude injection into any major vessels (aorta) or into the psoas muscle and lumbar plexus (Figure 8.1). A solution of 10 mL of 1% lidocaine is injected (sometimes with long-acting steroids). A neurolytic block may be used for malignant pain or end stage peripheral vascular disease as 5–6 mL of 6% aqueous phenol. The ipsilateral extremity will feel warm if the block is successful. In neurolytic blocks pain improvement can be immediate or may take 24–48 hours to be complete. In other conditions, pain can initially increase.

8.8.2 Complications and side effects

Hypotension is an immediate side effect especially if bilateral blocks are done. More serious long-term complications are aortitis (intra-aortic injection), motor block (posterior spread to the nerve roots or even epidurally), impotence or neuropathic pain often in the genito-femoral area (15% of patients report some neuropathic pain after neurolytic block).

8.8.3 Benefits and repeatability

Neurolytic blocks are rarely repeated.

8.9 Coeliac plexus block and renal nerve block

Visceral pain arising from the pancreas or kidneys can be difficult to treat with opioids alone. Afferent nociceptive fibres from the viscera accompany the sympathetic nerves. A sympathetic block interrupts these pathways and also the viscero-visceral reflexes that cause is-chaemia and spasm.

8.10 Coeliac plexus block (anterocrural approach)

8.10.1 Indications

- Acute pain, performed during surgery for postoperative pain relief
- Chronic severe upper abdominal visceral pain such as chronic pancreatitis (local anaesthetic blocks only).

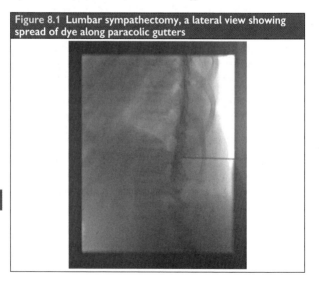

Figure 8.1 Lumbar sympathectomy, a lateral view showing spread of dye along paracolic gutters

- Upper abdominal organ cancer pain, frequently used for carcinoma of the pancreas, where an initial diagnostic local anaesthetic is followed by a neurolytic block can. A recent CT scan should be available.

8.10.2 Contraindications

- Grossly abnormal coagulopathy
- Anatomical complications such as a large thoraco-abdominal aneurysm, malignancy invading the retroperitoneal space.

8.10.3 Technique

Sedation and intravenous fluids are required; the block is either performed under X-ray or CT guidance. The posterior approach is preferred with the patient placed prone. Bilateral insertion of needle (e.g. 20G 20-cm needles) anterior to the body of L1 vertebrae (Figure 8.2), with entry point 6–8 cm lateral avoiding lung, kidneys and major vessels. The needle is advanced anteriorly, medially and cranially hitting the bony L1 body and checking in a lateral view to slide the needle forward so it comes to rest anterior to the vertebral body. Confirmation with radio opaque contrast is essential to confirm paracoelic spread and exclude intravascular placement, injection into the aortic wall or posterior spread.

Figure 8.2 End points for posterior approach to the coeliac plexus

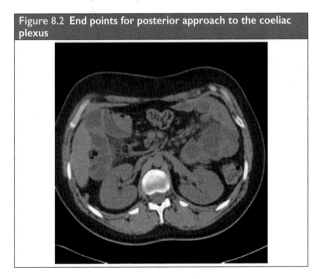

Figure 8.2 CT cross section at L1 visualizing end point of needle placement in coeliac plexus, passing below the 12th rib and 7 cm from midline of spinous process on either side of the L1 vertebral body.

Initial diagnostic blocks are performed with local anaesthetic, prior to any neurolytic blocks; the latter are almost always done in the palliative setting. Diagnostic and therapeutic local anaesthetic injections may be performed with up to 20 mL of plain lidocaine 1% or bupivacaine 0.25%. Depot preparations of steroid can be added for chronic pancreatitis. For a neurolytic block alcohol is the agent of choice, and up to 50 mL of alcohol 50–75% is injected on each side; neat alcohol is diluted with either bupivacaine 0.25% or lidocaine 1%. The addition of contrast confirms adequate spread. Phenol (usually 6%) can be used in smaller volumes of 5–10 mL per side, but it is best targeted at the greater splanchnic nerves as only such a low volume is possible for toxicity reasons. Its immediate local anaesthetic effect obviates any pain on injection (Eisenberg et al., 1995, Mercadante et al., 1998).

8.10.4 Special points

Complications include rapid absorption of agent, leading to systemic toxicity, possible subarachnoid injection, and sympathetic blockade leading to decreased blood pressure, often seen as orthostatic hypotension. Bleeding, infection, aortic dissection, pneumothorax and puncture of the kidney are possible. With neurolytic blocks the patient has to be informed about diarrhoea, sexual dysfunction and paraplegia.

8.10.5 Benefits and repeatability

The benefit of sympathetic anaesthetic block is still under discussion and there are new approaches endoscopically that have less serious potential complications. However, patients with pancreatic cancer have better pain relief after a neurolytic block than with systemic analgesic therapy alone.

Neurolytic coeliac plexus block (NCPB) in the palliative setting produces 85% success. 70–80% patients report almost immediate pain relief and in 60–75% this lasts until death; 90% report reduction in opioid use. NCPB offers both analgesic and non-analgesic benefits, such as increased alertness and limitation of drug systemic side effects. It is especially efficacious if used early and may require a repeat injection in patients with prolonged survival.

NCPB in chronic pancreatitis is transiently effective in 50–70% of patients, probably due to scarring and fibrosis. CPB using local anaesthetics is preferred in this condition, where pain relief, if any, can last 2–4 months and the risks are greatly reduced.

8.11 Renal nerve block

This unilateral sympathetic block at L1 has been used with chronic pain; there is some limited efficacy in patients suffering from haematuria loin pain syndrome. Local anaesthetic alone or with a long-acting steroid is injected under imaging. The procedure is similar to a unilateral coeliac plexus block in terms of technique and risks.

8.12 **Hypogastric block**

Indications for this uncommon block are pelvic visceral pain and refractory testicular pain. Optimal results require fluoroscopic identification of the triangle formed by shadows of the L5 transverse process, sacral and iliac crest.

8.13 **Ganglion impar block**

Indications are diagnostic and therapeutic management of sympathetically mediated pain of the perineum, rectum and genitalia. It can also be used in malignancy, endometriosis and proctalgia fugax. The terminal paravertebral sympathetic chain receives fibres from both lumbar and sacral sympathetic and parasympathetic systems. A spinal needle is placed anterior to the sacrococcygeal junction under fluoroscopy. Complications include rectal perforation, fistula formation, epidural spread, and periosteal injection.

8.14 **Joint injections**

8.14.1 **Cervical facet joint injections (CFJI)**

CFJI can be useful in neck pain in degenerative disease or in non-radicular pain radiating down the arms with normal neurology. Diagnostic or therapeutic injections in post-laminectomy pain can be used to confirm origins of pain.

Technique

The patient is positioned supine with arms down on the affected side. Under fluoroscopy the facet joints are visualized in the lateral view. The eye of the 'Scottie dog' is generally the point of the posterior branch of medial nerve and the facets are located slightly medial and posterior. The side to be injected is viewed as an oblique for better visualization using a locator. With a 25G needle the facets are approached inline with the radiation beam. The final position has to be checked and after negative aspiration 1–2 mL of mixture injected. Multiple facet blocks can be performed in one session.

8.14.2 **Thoracic facet joint injections (TFJI)**

TFJI is indicated for thoracic facet joint pain and very tender paravertebral points on palpation. The patient is prone and location of facet joints is similar to in the lumbar area. It can be difficult to inject into the facet joints here as they are small and peri-articular injection is often used.

8.14.3 **Lumbar facet joint injections (LFJI)**

LFJI are used for diagnostic and therapeutic purposes in the treatment of chronic mechanical back pain which can be accompanied by pain in buttocks and thighs, not normally extending below the knees (Carette *et al.*, 1991). The facet joints are often tender to palpation and extension androtation limited. Neurological examination is normal. Often there is no correlation between the radiological appearance and intensity of pain.

Technique

The patient is prone with a pillow cushioning the stomach to reduce the lumbar lordosis. The facet joint is located in the AP and oblique views (Figure 8.3). 1–2 mL of solution is injected at the required levels; multiple levels may be injected.

8.14.4 **Sacroiliac joint injection (SIJI)**

The patient is prone. The SI joint is located by AP fluoroscopy, but the obliquity of the view is to the opposite side to injected side. This is to avoid the iliac crest obscuring the view.

8.14.5 **Medial branch nerve denervation of facet joints**

Indications

This may be performed for patients with lumbar facet joint pain, hip and buttock pain, cramping lower extremity pain, lower back stiffness in absence of radiological disc herniation, spinal stenosis or foraminal

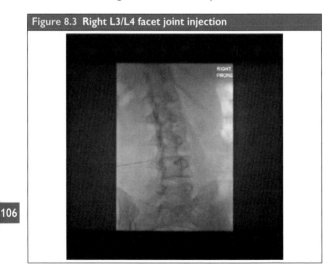

Figure 8.3 Right L3/L4 facet joint injection

root impingement. Any destructive lesioning should only follow successful diagnostic medial branch block with local anaesthetic.

Technique

Fluoroscopy is performed at the target point with minimum oblique to visualize the eye of 'Scottie dog'; the probe tip position is viewed in multiplane views before negative aspiration and injection of local anaesthetic and steroid.

Special points

The posterior medial branch can be denervated with a similar procedure to lumbar facet block except aiming for the 'eye of the Scottie dog'. Performing radiofrequency-pulsed lesions following a positive diagnostics block is possible after two successful diagnostic injections.

Complications

Transient increase in pain, aspiration of blood or CSF, Charcot joint pain due to denervation after radiofrequency can all occur.

Benefits and repeatability

Recent studies suggest that whether or not the injection is actually in the facet joint makes little difference immediately or long term. Short-lived success (less than 6 weeks) with local anaesthetic and steroid is said to be improved by use of radiofrequency lesions to the nerves to the joints.

8.14.6 Intra-articular injection

Intra-articular joint injections were first introduced in 1950s and are a good treatment for musculoskeletal conditions that are frequently performed by rheumatologists, orthopaedic surgeons and primary care physicians.

Primary indications are inflammatory spondyloarthropathies, although osteoarthritic conditions have also been anecdotally treated successfully. Shoulder, elbow, knee and hips joints are commonly injected. The main principles are to use a clean technique and to use the smallest possible needle (25G) to gain access to the area of maximal tenderness. Ultrasound has been used in locating the exact point; however, per-articular injections have been shown to be beneficial. In bursitis, if a bursa is palpable then injection directly into it is advocated. Steroids and local anaesthetics are the solutions in frequent use. Hyaluronic acid, a naturally occurring substance in synovial joint, has been used but the evidence is not well validated. These injections should be limited to a maximum of three a year as they tend to be less efficacious over time.

8.15 **Peripheral nerve blocks**

Only specific chronic pain related peripheral nerve blocks will be described.

8.15.1 **Selective nerve root blocks**

Indications

Root nerve blocks can be a useful diagnostic tool in the assessment of back pain. In patients with radicular symptoms with equivocal clinical and radiological imaging, a root block can help to determine the source of the symptoms. The procedure is therefore often curative. In post-discectomy pain and pain after disc herniation, a root nerve block can provide excellent analgesia and surgery can sometimes be avoided (Slosar & White 1998).

General contraindications

Infection locally or systemically, impaired coagulation and severe canal stenosis.

Technique

A nerve stimulator is used; to ensure adequate distance from the nerve there should be no stimulation below 0.3 mA. Negative aspiration and the use of contrast while screening are also important. If the needle has been properly placed, the contrast will flow around the nerve root and may cause radicular pain correlating with the patient's usual pain pattern.

8.15.2 **Cervical nerve root block**

Technique

The patient is supine with arms by the sides, it may be necessary to pull on the arms to obtain clear view of cervical spine. X-ray is used in the lateral view to locate intervertebral foraminae. The entry point is usually about 5 cm from the midline, aiming the needle medially and caudally towards the posterior vertebral foraminal border, hitting the bone and then walking caudally off the bone until the foraminal space is located. AP views are taken to ensure that the depth of needle is appropriate and not beyond the midline. Less than 2 mL of solution is needed per nerve root.

8.15.3 **Thoracic nerve root block**

Technique

The patient is prone with the arms hanging over the table edge to rotate scapulae out of the way. The C arm of the image intensifier is placed in the AP plane. The intervertebral foramen is located, and the head of rib is identified. The needle entry point is below the caudal edge of rib about 5 cm from the midline. The needle is aimed towards the vertebral lamina hitting the bone and is then walked off laterally. There may be a 'give' as needle enters the foramen. The needle should not be advanced more than to an imaginary line joining the facet joints in the midline. The C arm is then rotated to obtain a lateral view, ensuring the needle lies in the posterior aspect of foramen.

8.15.4 **Lumbar nerve root block**

Technique

The patient is prone with a pillow under the abdomen to help reduce the lumbar lordosis. The C arm is in the AP view to locate the transverse process adjacent to intervertebral foramen of interest. The needle entry point is at the tip of the transverse process about 2 cm caudally and 5 cm from the midline aiming for the vertebral lamina and walking off its posterior wall into the foramen. An alternate method is to aim for the transverse process and walk the needle off the process caudally and sliding off medially (Figure 8.4).

8.15.5 **Sacral nerve root block (SNRB) S1 and S2, 3, 4**

Technique

The technique for blocking the S1 nerve root is governed by the different anatomy of the sacrum and its foramina. The S1 nerve roots course medial to the S1 pedicle before leaving the sacrum through the S1 anterior sacral foramen which lies below and lateral to the pedicle. The target point for an S1 block lies at the inferior medial

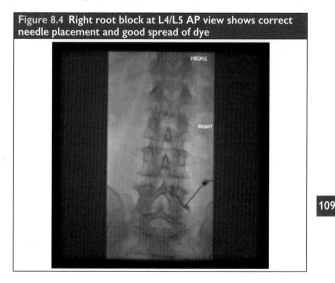

Figure 8.4 Right root block at L4/L5 AP view shows correct needle placement and good spread of dye

corner of the pedicle and access to this point is obtained through the posterior sacral foramen. A 22G spinal needle should be inserted through the skin behind the sacrum lateral and below the target point on the S1 pedicle. The objective is to have the tip of the needle rest on the medial end of the caudal surface of the pedicle behind the anterior wall of the sacrum. To achieve this position, the needle must pass through the posterior sacral foramen but must not leave the sacrum through the anterior sacral foramen.

End points
The needle 'walks' down the superior wall of the foramen which is formed by the S1. Passage through the anterior sacral foramen will be indicated by loss of resistance, in which case the needle should be withdrawn and replaced in contact with the pedicle. Blocking the S2–S4 nerves is essentially done through the sacral hiatus (effectively a caudal block).

Complications and side effects
Immediate complications can be aspiration of blood or CSF. Pneumothorax can occur in cervical and thoracic RNB. The patient should always be warned of the possibility of increase in pain and the side effects from steroids.

Evidence
Nerve root blocks are very effective in the non-operative treatment of minor mono-radiculopathy and should be recommended as the initial treatment of choice for this condition. There is no definitive research to dictate the frequency of SNRBs, it is generally considered reasonable to limit SNRBs to three times per year.

8.16 Nerve blocks for headaches

Occipital and C2 selective nerve block and greater and lesser occipital nerve blocks can be useful in this patient population. Trigeminal nerve blocks are of particular use in trigeminal neuralgia.

8.17 Central blocks

8.17.1 Epidural blockade
Epidural steroid injections can play a part in the non-surgical management of lumbar radicular pain and cervical radiculopathy.

Technique
The patient is positioned lateral or prone, sedation, IV access and IV fluids may be necessary. Fluoroscopy is essential to confirm needle position in the epidural space (up to 13% of injections can be outside the space). A standard epidural loss of resistance technique to saline

or air will identify the epidural space; however, an epidurogram under fluoroscopy is needed to confirm epidural spread (Figure 8.5).

Benefits and repeatability

Conventional epidural injection of steroids can be described as a 'general' approach, covering many spinal levels but administering only a small amount of steroid at each level. A selective nerve root block is more of a 'target' approach, with the injection of a relatively high dose of steroid around a specific nerve root.

8.17.2 **Epiduroscopy**

Epiduroscopy (myeloscopy, spinoscopy) was developed in 1990. A fibre optic camera is inserted percutaneously through the sacral hiatus, and is then guided upwards towards the lower lumbar discs and nerve roots. It is minimally invasive diagnostic and therapeutic procedure (Igarashi et al., 2004).

Indications

Epidural adhesions can usually be identified on an enhanced MRI scan using intravenous gadolinium. As some adhesions can prevent epidurally injected drugs from reaching the inflamed nerve roots, this technique can be used to treat inflamed nerve roots when epidural injections/nerve root blocks have been unsuccessful. It is particularly useful in elderly patients with degenerative spinal stenosis and radiculopathy; epidural adhesions can be released, e.g. post-disc surgery or with inflammatory radicular pain.

Contraindications

Special considerations in patients with raised intracranial pressure.

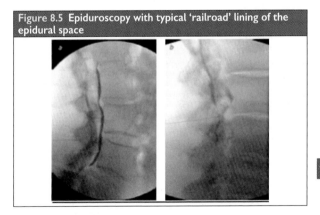

Figure 8.5 Epiduroscopy with typical 'railroad' lining of the epidural space

Technique

Sedation may be necessary; a sterile technique is used under image intensifier guidance with a flexible fibre optic catheter. The patient is positioned prone. The epidural space is accessed using a Seldinger wire inserted through a caudally placed needle. After the dilator sheath is inserted, the epiduroscope is passed. Success depends on the skill of the operator and the underlying pathology. The benefits may take weeks or months to develop.

Complications and side effects

Residual pain and numbness at insertion site, bowel, bladder and sexual dysfunction have been reported. Technical problems, e.g. difficulty passing scope or scope breakage, and infection.

8.17.3 Intradiscal electrothermal therapy (IDET)

IDET is a minimally invasive outpatient surgical procedure developed to treat patients with chronic low back pain that is caused by tears or small hernias of lumbar discs. Therefore, it is mainly for patients with discogenic pain resistant to aggressive non-surgical intervention.

Discography, a provocative test, piercing the disc with a thin needle and injecting a contrast, is used to identify the painful disc by provoking pain in the affected disc. This also shows whether the dye leaks out of an annular tear.

Indications

- Small hernias
- Internal disc tears
- Mild disc degeneration limited to one or two levels.

Contraindications

- Severe disc degeneration
- Spinal stenosis
- Neurological symptoms (such as leg weakness)
- Large disc herniations
- Requires a well-sedated patient as it is minimally invasive surgery but verbal contact should be maintained.

Technique

The patient is positioned prone. The procedure is performed with fluoroscopy and requires local anaesthetic and minimal intravenous sedation. A hollow introducer needle is inserted into the painful lumbar disc space using fluoroscopy. An electrothermal catheter (heating wire) is then passed through the needle and positioned along the disc annulus. The catheter tip is then slowly heated to

90°C for 15–17 minutes. The heat contracts and thickens the collagen fibres in the disc wall, promoting closure of the tears and cracks. Tiny nerve endings are cauterized, making them less sensitive.

Special points

A lumbar support is worn for 6–8 weeks, followed by an appropriate course of physical therapy. Lifting and bending precautions are necessary during this time to allow for adequate healing of the disc.

Complications and side effects

Nerve damage in less than 1%; damage and infection of the disc have been reported.

Evidence

This is a relatively new procedure and the evidence is equivocal. There is a need for more trials of good quality; however, this is limited by the highly selective group of patients required to show marginal benefit.

8.17.4 **Vertebroplasty**

Percutaneous vertebroplasty may be used to provide pain relief for patients with severe painful osteoporosis, loss of height, compression fractures or symptomatic painful vertebral body tumours. It can be done under sedation with local anaesthetic. It involves the injection of acrylic bone cement into the vertebral body via a trocar guided by fluoroscopy. This can relieve pain, stabilize the fractured vertebrae and in some cases, restore vertebral height (straightening out the spinal curve). Kyphoplasty is similar to vertebroplasty; however, an inflatable balloon device is inserted into the vertebra through the needle. As the balloon is inflated, it opens up a space that is then filled with the bone cement. Extrusion of cement is a real risk. These procedures are done by either interventional radiologists or orthopaedic surgeons in the UK.

8.17.5 **Interspinous Process Distractor (X–STOP)**

The X-STOP is an interspinous implant for patients whose symptoms are exacerbated in spinal extension and relieved in flexion. It has been available in Europe since June 2002. X-STOP is mainly indicated in patients with spinal stenosis who have unrelieved symptoms with aggressive medical management, and the only option available is surgery. It can be performed under sedation with local anaesthetic and involves the implantation of a titanium device between the spinous ligaments forcing the spine into a flexed position and alleviating lateral recess stenosis. Early trials suggest comparable symptomatic relief to laminectomy but with lower morbidity.

8.17.6 **Intrathecal drug delivery (ITDD)**

This method of drug delivery allows modulation of pain transmission at the spinal cord receptors conferring highly selective spinal analgesia, with fewer side effects than after systemic agents. The agents used intrathecally have been reviewed and an international consensus algorithm is in place for drug choices based on safety, efficacy and clinical data. It supports the first-line use of morphine and hydromorphone and ziconotide (Deer *et al.*, 2007). Intra-cerebroventricular infusions of morphine have been used in patients with intractable head and neck cancer pain and seem to provide some pain relief; however, more clinical data are necessary before this can be widely advocated.

Indications

- Chronic non-cancer pain which is unresponsive to other analgesia or when analgesia leads to intolerable side effects
- Cancer pain that is uncontrolled with appropriate systemic opioids or when these give intolerable side effects
- Spasticity.

Contraindications

- Raised intracranial pressure, impending cord compression
- Allergy to specific medication used
- Factors that may affect surgical risk include haematological derangement, wound infections, emaciation and the presence of tumours in the spinal canal
- Poor patient compliance
- Lack of local expertise
- Lack of support services for ongoing care.

Pre-procedure considerations

Patients need to be carefully selected within a multidisciplinary setting preferably with a comprehensive psychological assessment. Preoperative systemic drugs should be converted to short acting drugs, reducing the risk of withdrawal symptoms. The device has to be carefully chosen and the site of implantation of pump reservoir, type and refill intervals identified.

Technique

The patient is placed lateral with good access to the spine and abdomen.

The intrathecal catheter is placed using a posterior midline approach and fed to the desired level under fluoroscopy. The catheter can either tunnelled to an external pump (with suitable filters) or it can be connected to a fully implanted pump placed surgically in the subcutaneous layer of the abdomen.

Special points
Several different types of drug delivery systems are available:
- Percutaneous catheters (tunnelled or not) used with an external pump, which are easy to place, good if patient has limited life expectancy of less than 3 months; however, they restrict mobility.
- Totally implantable systems with subcutaneous injection port connected to external pump may be preferred for longer term use.
- Fully implantable ITDD systems provide maximum mobility and functional activity.

Complications
- Drug related and specific to each agent
- Catheter related
  - Immediate: Dural puncture headache, nerve damage, haematoma
  - Late: catheter-related inflammatory mass, infection, catheter migration or breakage
- Delivery system: Pump failure or refill/programming errors. Malfunction can occur with internal systems in MRI scanners. Internal devices need to be removed post mortem prior to cremation.

Evidence
In many cases, the initial high costs of a totally implanted ITDD system are recovered by 28 months compared with conventional therapy.

8.17.7 Spinal cord stimulation (SCS)
SCS probably acts by directly inhibiting the transmission of pain in the dorsal horn of the spinal cord and promoting descending brain and spinal inhibition.

Indications (See Box 8.1).

Contraindications
Absolute contraindications: Demand-type cardiac pacemaker, implanted cardiac defibrillator, uncontrolled coagulopathy and sepsis.

Technique
The patient may require some sedation for this procedure but verbal contact is vital when trying to position the SCS lead. A sterile theatre environment is mandatory due to the risk of infection. It is prudent administer antibiotics prophylactically due to risk of infection with *Staphylococcus aureus*. The patient is positioned initially prone for placement of the electrode(s), followed by a lateral position to implant the impulse generator in the anterior abdominal wall. Initially, the electrodes are placed into the posterior epidural space percutaneously via a needle. Pelvic pain may be treated by retrograde lead

Box 8.1 Indications for SCS

Good indications for SCS (good response)
- Neuropathic pain in limb following lumbar or cervical spine surgery
- Complex regional pain syndrome
- Neuropathic pain secondary to peripheral nerve damage
- Pain associated with peripheral vascular disease
- Refractory angina
- Some visceral pains.

Intermediate indications for SCS (may respond)
- Amputation pain (stump pain responds better than phantom pain)
- Axial pain following spinal surgery
- Intercostal neuralgia, e.g. post-thoracotomy or post-herpetic neuralgia
- Pain associated with spinal cord damage
- Peripheral neuropathic pain syndromes.

Poor indications for SCS (rarely respond)
- Central pain of non-spinal cord origin
- Spinal cord injury with clinically complete loss of posterior column function
- Plexus complete avulsions.

insertion to stimulate sacral roots. Surgically placed electrodes can also be used. The position of the electrodes determines the distribution of the paraesthesiae that must cover the area of pain by at least 80% if the technique is to be effective. There is controversy about the value of trial stimulation as a predictor of long-term success.

Side effects
- Bleeding
- Nerve damage or paralysis
- Pain around the implant site
- Lead fractures and the need for re-operation
- Unable to undergo MRI investigations.

8.18 Deep brain stimulation (DBS) and motor cortex stimulation (MCS)

Satisfactory pain relief can be achieved in patients with intractable chronic neuropathic pain, central thalamic pain and post stroke pain syndromes as the stimulation site is moved to higher levels. This implies that abnormal processing of nociceptive information develops at the level of deafferentation and spreads rostrally. Electrodes for

DBS are implanted within the periventricular grey matter, specific sensory thalamic nuclei or the internal capsule; DBS may increase the concentrations of the inhibitory neurotransmitter glutamate.

MCS utilizes evoked potentials specific to the painful area to confer a state of inhibition thereby providing some pain relief; this effect is short-lived.

Both of these methods require neurosurgical expertise and are only appropriate in a small subset of patients, this limits the availability of meaningful clinical research data.

8.19 Conclusion

Interventional techniques provide a useful tool for diagnosing and treating pain syndromes. They have a place within a multidisciplinary pain management approach. However, the overall functional rehabilitation of the patient is an important goal. The integration of physical and psychological support is essential for this to be achieved.

Key references

Alvarez D, Rockwell PG (2002). Trigger points: diagnosis and management. *Am. Fam. Physician* **65**: 4.

Carette S, Marcoux S, Truchon R, *et al.* (1991). A controlled trial of corticosteroid injections into facet joints for chronic low back pain. *New Engl. J. Med.* **325**: 1002–7.

Eichenberger U, Greher M, Curatolo M (2004). Ultrasound in interventional pain management. *Tech. Reg. Anesth. Pain Manag.* **8**: 171–8.

Deer T, Krames ES, Hassenbusch SJ *et al.* Polyanalgesic Consensus Conference 2007: Recommendations for the Management of Pain by Intrathecal (Intraspinal) Drug Delivery: Report of an Interdisciplinary Expert Panel. Neuromodulation 2007; **10**: 300–28.

Eisenberg E, Carr DB, Chalmers TC (1995). Neurolytic celiac plexus block for treatment of cancer pain: a meta-analysis. *Anesth. Analg.* **80**: 290–5.

Erickson SJ, Hogan QH (1993). CT-guided injection of the stellate ganglion: description of technique and efficacy of sympathetic blockade. *Radiology* **188**: 707–9.

Igarashi T, Hirabayashi Y, Seo N, Saitoh K, Fukuda H, Suzuki H (2004). Lysis of adhesions and epidural injection of steroid/local anaesthetic during epiduroscopy potentially alleviate low back and leg pain in elderly patients with lumbar spinal stenosis. *Br. J. Anaesth.* **93**: 181–7.

Mercadante S, Nicosia F (1998). Coeliac plexus block: a reappraisal. *Reg. Anesth. Pain Med.* **23**: 37–48.

Slosar PJ, White AH (1998). The use of selective nerve root blocks: diagnostic, therapeutic, or placebo? *Spine* **23**: 2253–4.

Chapter 9

Non-pharmacological approaches to pain management

Mark I. Johnson and Jan M. Bjordal

Key points

- TENS, acupuncture and physiotherapy have a key role within multimodal management of chronic pain. Physiotherapy interventions include manipulation, mobilization, massage, exercise and low level laser therapy
- Repeated treatment is required because effects are generally short-term, although they have low toxicity, are generally safe and can be used in combination with other interventions
- Trained specialists are required to administer acupuncture and physiotherapy. TENS and exercise can be administered by the patient themselves
- Systematic reviews have shown these treatments to be superior to non-treatment and to sham interventions, although the findings have been challenged due to methodological shortcomings
- Head-to-head comparisons with other non-pharmacological treatments often show equivalence of effect so treatment choice is made on a case by case basis.

9.1 Transcutaneous electrical nerve stimulation (TENS)

TENS is a non-invasive technique whereby pulsed electrical currents generated by a battery powered stimulating device are passed across the surface of the skin to stimulate underlying nerves (Figure 9.1). Patients self-administer TENS and titrate the dosage of treatment as required. TENS effects are often immediate with few side effects and

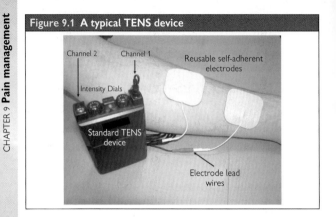

Figure 9.1 A typical TENS device

Channel 2   Channel 1   Reusable self-adherent electrodes

Intensity Dials

Standard TENS device

Electrode lead wires

no potential for toxicity. TENS devices are inexpensive (£30GBP) and can be purchased without medical prescription in some countries. A supervised trial of TENS and a point of contact to troubleshoot problems are recommended for new patients (Walsh, 1997).

9.1.1 Biological rationale and plausibility

The conventional way of administering TENS (conventional TENS) is to deliver currents in order to selectively activate large diameter non-noxious afferents (Aβ) without activating smaller diameter nociceptive afferents (Aδ and C). This inhibits ongoing activity in second-order nociceptive neurones in the spinal cord. A strong but non-painful TENS paraesthesia is indicative of non-noxious afferent (Aβ) activity (Figure 9.2). Another type of TENS, termed acupuncture like (AL-TENS), uses bursts (trains) of pulses to generate non-painful phasic muscle contractions and is used when patients do not respond to conventional TENS. The resultant small diameter muscle afferent activity activates descending pain inhibitory pathways. There are many 'TENS-like devices' available on the market including microcurrent stimulation, transcutaneous spinal electroanalgesia (TSE), interferential therapy (IFT) and Pain®Gone pens. There is a lack of good quality research evidence to support their use (Johnson, 2008).

9.1.2 Principles of use for conventional TENS

Electrode position

TENS electrodes must be positioned on healthy sensate skin. TENS electrodes are placed around the site of pain so that paraesthesia can be directed into the painful area for most types of pain. If tactile allodynia is present electrodes should be placed along nerves proximal to the site of pain in the first instance as TENS may aggravate the pain.

Electrodes can also be positioned paravertebrally at the appropriate spinal segment, or proximally in the same dermatome when electrode placement at the site of pain is not possible due to an open wound, or the absence of a limb (Figure 9.3a and 9.3b). Electrode placement in contralateral dermatomes is another option, but experimental studies suggest this electrode placement is less effective than the other options.

Electrical characteristics of TENS

The user titrates the intensity of TENS to generate a strong, comfortable, non-painful TENS paraesthesia beneath the electrodes. Theoretically, pulses delivered anywhere between 10 and 200 pulses per second using a continuous pulse pattern and pulse durations between 50 and 500 μs help to achieve this effect (Figure 9.4). In practice, patients are encouraged to experiment with TENS settings for pulse frequency, pulse pattern and pulse duration because optimal settings remain unknown.

Timing and dosage

TENS effects are maximal during stimulation so patients should leave electrodes *in situ* and administer TENS intermittently throughout the day. Minor skin irritation may occur so users should attend to skin care underneath the electrodes and change electrode positions if skin irritation is bothersome. The onset of relief is often immediate. Reports of the duration of post-treatment effects vary considerably.

Contraindications and precautions

TENS should not be used on patients with cardiac pacemakers or a history of cardiac problems without prior discussion with their cardiologist. TENS should not be administered over the abdomen during pregnancy because currents could inadvertently cause uterine contractions and the effects of TENS on foetal development are not known. TENS should not be applied on the head or neck of patients with epilepsy, and not given to patients with compromised circulation such as thrombosis. Electrodes should not be applied internally,

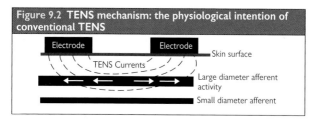

Figure 9.2 TENS mechanism: the physiological intention of conventional TENS

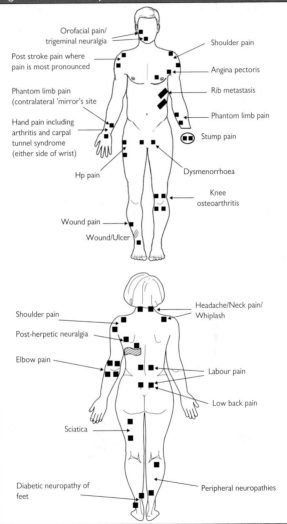

Figure 9.3 Electrode placement for TENS

Orofacial pain/ trigeminal neuralgia

Shoulder pain

Post stroke pain where pain is most pronounced

Angina pectoris

Phantom limb pain (contralateral 'mirror's site

Rib metastasis

Phantom limb pain

Hand pain including arthritis and carpal tunnel syndrome (either side of wrist)

Stump pain

Hp pain

Dysmenorrhoea

Knee osteoarthritis

Wound pain

Wound/Ulcer

Shoulder pain

Headache/Neck pain/ Whiplash

Post-herpetic neuralgia

Elbow pain

Labour pain

Low back pain

Sciatica

Diabetic neuropathy of feet

Peripheral neuropathies

Figure 9.3 is reproduced from Bennett, M. (2006). *Neuropathic Pain*, pp. 120, with permission from Oxford University Press.

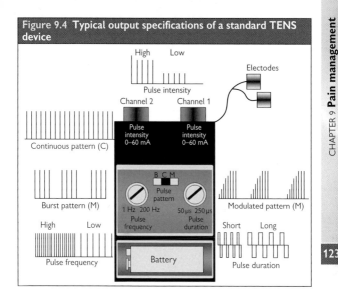

Figure 9.4 Typical output specifications of a standard TENS device

High   Low

Electrodes

Pulse intensity

Channel 2   Channel 1

Pulse intensity 0–60 mA

Pulse intensity 0–60 mA

Continuous pattern (C)

B C M

Pulse pattern

1 Hz 200 Hz   50 µs 250 µs

Pulse frequency   Pulse duration

Burst pattern (M)

Modulated pattern (M)

High   Low

Short   Long

Pulse frequency

Battery

Pulse duration

123

over damaged or insensate skin, on the anterior neck or close to transdermal drug delivery systems. TENS should not be used while operating hazardous equipment or motor vehicles but can be used whilst going to sleep providing the TENS device has a timer so that it automatically switches off. Children as young as four appear to be able to tolerate TENS treatment. Decisions are left to the discretion of the medical practitioner.

9.1.3 **Clinical effectiveness**

There are over 400 randomized controlled clinical trials (PubMed, 12 March 2007), although many have methodological shortcomings, including inappropriate TENS technique and under dosing. For this reason, systematic reviews and meta-analyses on TENS that are available as evidence are inconclusive for mixed populations of chronic pain patients, chronic lower back pain, rheumatoid arthritis of the hand, whiplash and mechanical neck disorders, post-stroke shoulder pain and chronic recurrent headache. One Cochrane review reported that TENS relieves pain and stiffness associated with knee osteoarthritis (Osiri et al., 2000; for a review, see Johnson, 2008).

Clinical experience suggests that TENS is potentially useful for any type of chronic pain including those of nociceptive, neuropathic and musculoskeletal origin. Non-randomized trials suggest many types of

Figure 9.4 is reproduced from Bennett, M. (2006). *Neuropathic Pain*, pp. 121, with permission from Oxford University Press.

pain have long-term benefit from daily use of TENS including LBP, osteoarthritis, localized muscle pain and neuropathic pains of peripheral origin such as post-herpetic and trigeminal neuralgias, amputation pain, entrapment neuropathies and radiculopathies. TENS may also benefit metastatic bone disease, pains caused by secondary deposits, pains due to nerve compression by a neoplasm and post-mastectomy and post-thoracotomy pains.

9.2 **Acupuncture**

Acupuncture involves inserting fine disposable steel needles (0.2–0.3 mm diameter) through the skin at selected points to stimulate underlying nerve and muscle tissue. Additional stimulation is produced by 'twirling' the needle or by passing mild currents through pairs of needles using an electrical stimulator (electroacupuncture) (Figure 9.5). Originally, acupuncture was believed to alter the flow of vital energies of life (Yin and Yang) along energy channels (meridians). Nowadays, many practitioners adopt a Western approach which involves diagnosis according to orthodox medicine (Filshie & White, 1997). Despite its widespread use, acupuncture continues to be a controversial treatment (Ernst, 2006).

9.2.1 **Biological rationale and plausibility**

Evidence for meridians is not convincing and claims that acupuncture points relate to nerve bundles, myofascial trigger points and perivascular plexi has been challenged. Evidence suggests that needling activates polymodal receptors and/or their afferents (Aδ and C) and this generates segmental and extrasegmental modulation of nociceptive input through the release of endogenous opioids via descending pain inhibitory pathways. Post-stimulation effects have been attributed to positive feedback neural circuitry in the mesolimbic region of the brain (Kawakita & Okada, 2006). Acupuncture also affects autonomic

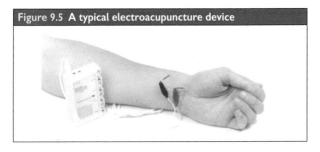

Figure 9.5 A typical electroacupuncture device

nervous system activity and improves microcirculation through axon reflexes and the release of vasoactive substances such as calcitonin gene-related peptide and substance P.

9.2.2 **Principles of use for manual acupuncture**

Point selection

Practitioners require formal training in acupuncture technique (www.medical-acupuncture.co.uk). Western practitioners use points from innervated regions according to known physiological principles, e.g. dermatome, myotome and sclerotome. Optimal point selection, the site and depth of needling is achieved through a careful process of trial and error. Patients sometimes report heaviness, soreness, dull ache, referred pain, numbness and/or paraesthesia during acupuncture. Stimulation of hyperaesthetic areas is avoided so needles are placed proximal to the site of nerve damage. Practitioners could stimulate above and below affected segments or use contralateral 'mirror' points in conditions like post-herpetic neuralgia or trigeminal neuralgia, or place needles to surround scars for phantom limb pain. Trigger points are used for pains of musculoskeletal origin. Stronger stimulation techniques are often used if distant points are chosen.

Timing and dosage

Needles are left in place for up to 30 minutes and manipulated 'twirl-ing' to facilitate stimulation. Pain relief often outlasts the period of needling by several days or weeks, although there may be a delay in onset with some patients experiencing an increase in pain in the first 48 hours. Pain relief may be cumulative over time with patients requiring 'top up' sessions. A typical course for a chronic condition could consist of 6–12 treatments given once per week.

Contraindications and precautions

Contraindications include needle phobia, bleeding disorders, antico-agulant medication and needling over a pregnant uterus. Electroacu-puncture is contraindicated for patients with cardiac pacemakers. Serious adverse events such as pneumothorax, cardiac tamponade and fatalities due to needle infection are very rare. Needle pain, tiredness, feeling faint and minor bleeding are more common.

9.2.3 **Clinical effectiveness**

There are over 900 randomized controlled clinical trials cited in PubMed (12 March 2007). Many have methodological shortcomings, although a more positive picture is emerging as better quality trials are published (Ernst, 2006). A systematic review of systematic reviews stated that there was no robust evidence that acupuncture works for any indication (Derry et al., 2006). This extreme view is not widely accepted because many systematic reviews have found evidence that acupuncture is superior to no treatment and/or sham acupuncture for chronic LBP, neck pain, chronic knee pain including knee osteoarthritis, peripheral joint osteoarthritis and fibromyalgia syndrome (Manheimer et al., 2005; White et al., 2007). Evidence is inconclusive for mixed populations of chronic pain and shoulder pain.

Clinical experience suggests that acupuncture is generally better for nociceptive and musculoskeletal pain than neuropathic pain. Nevertheless, benefit has been reported for phantom limb pain, diabetic neuropathy and neurogenic pruritus. Acupuncture seems promising in the short term for cancer pain but that there is a paucity of RCTs. Acupuncture may be worth a trial in a patient who has not responded to other treatments or who cannot tolerate drug therapy.

9.3 **Physiotherapy approaches**

Physiotherapists use a biopsychosocial model of pain and are well placed to improve chronic pain related disability by assessing pain, attitudes and beliefs, illness behaviour and the social environment. Physiotherapists require formal training (www.csp.org.uk). They have a variety of interventions and techniques at their disposal, including TENS and acupuncture, but detailed discussion lies outside the scope of this chapter. Systematic reviews suggests that pain-focused treatments are likely to have a positive impact on the chronic pain patient when used within a multidisciplinary pain management approach (Gifford et al., 2006).

9.3.1 **Clinical effectiveness**

Manipulation and mobilization

Evidence from systematic reviews is conflicting. Spinal manipulation was not effective as a stand-alone treatment for chronic LBP in one review but manipulation and mobilization was superior to general practitioner management in another (Bronfort et al., 2004). Manipulation and/or mobilization was not effective as a stand-alone treatment for chronic mechanical neck disorder but had short- and long-term benefits when combined with exercise (Gross et al., 2004). Spinal manipulation therapy was better than massage for cervicogenic headache.

Massage

Evidence from systematic reviews is inconclusive for massage as a stand-alone or multimodal treatment for neck pain (Ezzo et al., 2007) and for deep transverse friction massage for tendinitis pain.

Exercise

There is evidence for short-term benefits of specific stretching and strengthening exercises for chronic LBP, mechanical neck disorder, with or without headache, ankylosing spondylitis and rotator cuff disease (Smidt et al., 2005). McKenzie therapy, which treats LBP patients through individualized programmes of specific home exercises, has been shown to have short-term improvements in LBP when compared with other standard treatments and passive therapy (Clare *et al.*, 2004). The clinical relevance of the effect has been challenged.

Low level laser therapy (LLLT)

Systematic reviews provide evidence for short-term benefits from LLLT for chronic joint pain, chronic neck pain, adhesive capsulitis and rheumatoid arthritis, and that LLLT operates via an anti-inflammatory mechanism (Bjordal *et al.*, 2003, 2006; Chow & Barnsley, 2005; Figure 9.6). Evidence for osteoarthritis of the knee is conflicting due to variability in dosage and technique.

Other techniques

Spa therapy and balneotherapy may be effective for treating LBP. Evidence is inconclusive for traction in LBP or mechanical neck pain and for ultrasound in the treatment of musculoskeletal disorders. There is evidence that extracorporeal shock wave therapy (ESWT) provides no benefit in lateral elbow pain.

Supervised physiotherapy

Supervised group physiotherapy was better than home exercises, and combined inpatient spa-exercise therapy followed by supervised outpatient weekly group physiotherapy was better than weekly group physiotherapy alone (Dagfinrud *et al.*, 2005). Physical conditioning programmes supervised by physiotherapists are effective in reducing sick days for workers with chronic back pain when compared to usual care.

Figure 9.6 A typical low level laser therapy device

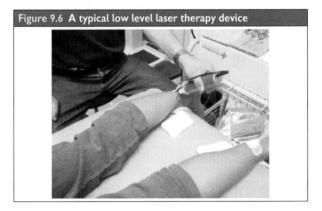

Evidence-based clinical practice guidelines

The Ottawa Panel recommends LLLT, ultrasound, thermotherapy, electrical stimulation and TENS for rheumatoid arthritis, and therapeutic exercises as a stand-alone treatment or combined with manual therapy for osteoarthritis (Ottawa Panel, 2005). The Philadelphia Clinical Practice Guideline Panel recommends normal activity for therapeutic exercise for chronic LBP; TENS and exercise for knee osteoarthritis; proprioceptive and therapeutic exercise for chronic neck pain; and the use of therapeutic ultrasound in the treatment of calcific tendonitis of the shoulder.

Key references

Bjordal JM, Couppe C, Chow RT, *et al.* (2003). A systematic review of low level laser therapy with location-specific doses for pain from chronic joint disorders. *Aust. J. Physiother.* **49**: 107–16.

Bjordal JM, Johnson MI, Iversen V, *et al.* (2006). Photoradiation in acute pain: a systematic review of possible mechanisms of action and clinical effects in randomized placebo-controlled trials. *Photomed. Laser Surg.* **24**: 158–68.

Bronfort G, Haas M, Evans RL, Bouter LM (2004). Efficacy of spinal manipulation and mobilization for low back pain and neck pain: a systematic review and best evidence synthesis. *Spine J.* **4**: 335–56.

Chow RT, Barnsley L (2005). Systematic review of the literature of low-level laser therapy (LLLT) in the management of neck pain. *Lasers Surg. Med.* **37**: 46–52.

Clare HA, Adams R, Maher CG (2004). A systematic review of efficacy of McKenzie therapy for spinal pain. *Aust. J. Physiother.* **50**: 209–16.

Dagfinrud H, Kvien TK, Hagen KB (2005). The Cochrane review of physiotherapy interventions for ankylosing spondylitis. *J. Rheumatol.* **32**: 1899–906.

Derry CJ, Derry S, McQuay HJ, Moore RA (2006). Systematic review of systematic reviews of acupuncture published 1996–2005. *Clin. Med.* **6**: 381–6.

Ernst E (2006). Acupuncture—a critical analysis. *J. Intern. Med.* **259**: 125–37.

Ezzo J, Haraldsson BG, Gross AR, *et al.* (2007). Massage for mechanical neck disorders: a systematic review. *Spine* **32**: 353–62.

Filshie J, White A (1997). *Medical Acupuncture: A Western Scientific Approach.* Churchill Livingstone, Edinburgh.

Gifford L, Thacker M, Jones MA (2006). Physiotherapy and pain. In SB MacMahon, M Koltzenburg (eds), *Textbook of Pain.* Elsevier, Philadelphia.

Gross AR, Hoving JL, Haines TA, *et al.* (2004). Manipulation and mobilisation for mechanical neck disorders. *Cochr. Database Syst. Rev.* CD004249.

Johnson MI. Transcutaneous electrical nerve stimulation. In T Watson (ed.), *Electrotherapy: Evidenced-Based Practice* 12th Edition Churchill Livingstone, Edinburgh 2008. Churchill Livingstone, Edinburgh.

Kawakita K, Okada K (2006). Mechanisms of action of acupuncture for chronic pain relief—polymodal receptors are the key candidates. *Acupunct. Med.* **24** (Suppl): S58–S66.

Manheimer E, White A, Berman B, *et al.* (2005). Meta-analysis: acupuncture for low back pain. *Ann. Intern. Med.* **142**: 651–63.

Osiri M, Welch V, Brosseau L, *et al.* (2000). Transcutaneous electrical nerve stimulation for knee osteoarthritis. *Cochr. Database Syst. Rev.* CD002823.

Ottawa Panel (2005). Ottawa panel evidence-based clinical practice guidelines for therapeutic exercises and manual therapy in the management of osteoarthritis. *Phys. Ther.* **85**: 907–71.

Smidt N, de Vet HC, Bouter LM, *et al.* (2005). Effectiveness of exercise therapy: a best-evidence summary of systematic reviews. *Aust. J. Physiother.* **51**: 71–85.

Walsh D (1997). *TENS. Clinical Applications and Related Theory*. Churchill Livingstone, New York.

White A, Foster NE, Cummings M, Barlas P (2007). Acupuncture treatment for chronic knee pain: a systematic review. *Rheumatology (Oxford)* **46**: 384–90.

Chapter 10

Psychological approaches to chronic pain

Stephen Morley

Key points

- Chronic pain has a significant interruptive effect: pain 'grabs' attention and has subtle influences on behaviour and cognition
- Chronic pain interferes with task performance and behavioural processes, particularly reinforcement will shape an individual's response to chronic pain
- Beliefs about pain and its consequences determine a person's adjustment to chronic pain and provide more explanatory variance that measures of pain *per se*
- A person's identity—there sense of who they are and their appraisal of their future self—is profoundly affected by chronic pain
- There is evidence that psychological treatments can be effective in moderating the impact of chronic pain on interruption, interference and identity.

10.1 Introduction

Chronic pain is more than a repeated or persistent experience of an intense, unpleasant sensation. It is frequently associated with widespread disruption of everyday behaviour, disengagement from normal social roles, e.g. work, exacerbated negative emotional states—particularly depression, frustration and anxiety, and subtle changes to a person's cognitive abilities such as memory and attention. The major tasks for the discipline of psychology are to develop scientifically testable models that account for the variations in the experience of people with persistent, difficult to treat pain and to devise treatments that can help ameliorate the range of suffering associated with pain. To a non-psychologist, the attempt to meet these objectives may often appear puzzling and the purpose of this chapter is to articulate a simple schematic framework into which some of the major issues can be accommodated. By way of analogy it may be helpful to think of a psychological cascade of processes that shape the range of experiences of people with chronic pain. The cascade may be conveniently schematized in a sequence of Interruption, Interference and impact of these on a person's Identity (Figure 10.1). Each of these components is briefly discussed and the chapter concludes with an overview of psychological treatments for chronic pain and a comment on their efficacy.

10.2 **Interruption**

A primary feature of pain is its capacity to interrupt ongoing behaviour on a moment-to-moment basis. The ability of pain signals to 'grab' attention is unrivalled and it demands that attention to be switched from its current focus to the experience of pain (Eccleston & Crombez, 1999; Crombez, 2006). Laboratory studies have used the primary task paradigm to model the interruptive effect of pain stimulus. In this task, participants engage in an attention demanding task such as a discrimination task, during which a painful stimulus is delivered. The interruptive effects of pain can be observed through the change in task performance. The effect of varying the pain parameters and primary task demands has been used to model the interruptive impact of pain. In laboratory studies, the extent of the interruption is a function of features of the pain such as the novelty, unpredictability, intensity and its threat value. There are two other potential sources of influence on the interruptive impact of pain:

- First, there are individual differences (traits) between people such as their fear of pain and there tendency to appraise the pain in a catastrophic manner. By their nature, it is difficult to manipulate these parameters experimentally but studies show a correlation between these features and the degree of interruption.

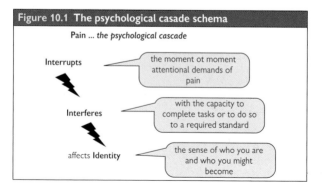

Figure 10.1 The psychological casade schema

Pain ... the psychological cascade

Interrupts — the moment ot moment attentional demands of pain

Interferes — with the capacity to complete tasks or to do so to a required standard

affects **Identity** — the sense of who you are and who you might become

- Second, the cognitive-affective model of pain suggests that attentional interruption is a function not only of the pain but also of the competing demands present in the current environment. Thus, in demanding environments the interruptive capacity of pain might be minimized while in undemanding environments pain may easily capture attention. So far, there are few experimental analyses of this hypothesis but observational studies provide supportive data, e.g. Beecher's famous observations on reduced reporting of pain by soldiers in the heat of battle. One implication of this is that chronic pain patients whose environment is limited through loss of important social roles, such as work, might be expected to be more vulnerable to the interruptive effects of pain

- Although experimental analyses of chronic pain is difficult, there is good evidence to show that the interruptive effects of pain are related to pain intensity and to individual differences such as catastrophizing. Moreover, the interruptive effect of chronic pain also affects the person's cognitive functioning so that subtle memory deficits may be present (Grisart & Van der Linden, 2001; Grisart et al., 2002).

10.3 **Interference**

Although acute pain may interrupt the execution of a task, it may still be possible to complete the task satisfactorily. However, repeated pain and interruption while executing a task may result in interference; that is, either failure to complete the task or a degradation of performance such that it is unsatisfactory when assessed against the person's implicit standards or another person's real or perceived demands (Pincus & Morley, 2001). It is the interference and threat of interference with behaviour that has the most visible impact on the pain sufferer. Interference is reflected in the extent of disability assessed by measures such as Pain Disability Index (Chibnall & Tait, 1994) and Sickness Impact Profile (Follick et al., 1985). The effect of interference in daily life is also seen in the high levels of frustration frequently reported by chronic pain patients.

This reduction in performance has been the subject of considerable analysis. Principles of operant learning theory (behavioural analysis) have been used to account for the development of behavioural patterns associated with pain (Sanders, 2002). Behaviour analysis identifies pain reduction as a potent source of negative reinforcement. The removal or reduction in intensity of a negative reinforcer increases the frequency (likelihood of occurrence) behaviours that precede it. Thus, pain reduction can reinforce rest, postural adjustment and the use of prosthetic aids, e.g. walking stick. This class of behaviours is generally referred to as pain behaviour. Positive reinforcement may also shape and maintain pain behaviour. Positive reinforcers are events which when presented increase the frequency (likelihood) of behaviours that precede them. A common class of positive reinforcement is the attention, concern and sympathy paid by significant others. Finally, behavioural analysis notes that certain contexts may exert discriminative control over a person's behaviour. For example, people may be more likely to complain of pain and to display a variety of pain behaviours in health care settings because such settings are associated with the occurrence of particular reinforcers. This analysis suggests that the degree of interference is not merely a function of pain intensity, frequency or duration, but it is shaped and developed by various environmental contingencies. It also provides the theoretical basis for behavioural interventions included in many treatment programmes.

Further evidence has accrued to show that *beliefs* about the experience of chronic pain are associated with adjustment to chronic pain. These studies are necessarily correlational and rely on statistical methods to demonstrate that the influence of pain is relatively less than the influence of beliefs about the impact of the pain (e.g. Crombez *et al.*, 1999); thus, providing the empirical basis for cognitive therapy. The cognitive mediation hypothesis has been elaborated in detail for a specific subgroup of people characterized by a specific cognitive mediator. In the fear-avoidance model of pain (Vlaeyen & Linton, 2000), which is shown diagrammatically in Figure 10.2, the crucial element is that catastrophic thoughts related to fear that making certain movements may lead to physical harm. This results in marked avoidance of activity and the perseveration of fear governed by the same mechanisms that are found in other fear related disorders (phobias). This model suggests that effective treatment should follow the principles of graded exposure to the feared events (Vlaeyen *et al.*, 2002). Further detailed cognitive models are currently being developed to account for a sub-group of patients in whom overuse rather than avoidance is associated with pain (Vlaeyen & Morley, 2004; Hasenbring *et al.*, 2006).

10.4 **Identity**

Both interruption and interference have unwanted behavioural, cognitive and emotional consequences but these may be relatively transient. Repeated interference has, however, a more significant impact on a person's abilities to engage with their major life goals and effectively disrupts their sense of self. Evidence for this comes from qualitative studies that have analysed individuals' accounts of living with chronic pain (e.g. Kotarba, 1983; Osborn & Smith, 1998; Contrada & Ashmore, 1999). Although various analytic methods have been used, several themes consistently emerge (Table 10.1). These aspects of identity have an impact on a person's goals and aspirations. For example, a middle-aged person might inappropriately hope to regain the physical prowess of a man 15 years younger if he recovers from his chronic condition. More recently, quantitative methods have been developed to investigate the relationship between chronic pain, the sense of self and emotional adjustment (Morley et al., 2005).

If pain cannot be eliminated then a significant question for any individual is 'how can I lead a valued life in the presence of pain'. To do this might involve re-prioritizing or even abandoning a significant goal that many chronic pain patients hold onto: the pursuit of pain relief (Aldrich et al., 2000; De Vlieger et al., 2006). Unsurprisingly, this represents a significant challenge for many chronic pain patients, their families and health professionals alike. Nevertheless, a psychological treatment—acceptance and commitment therapy (ACT)—has been developed that can address these issues (McCracken et al., 2004; McCracken, 2005).

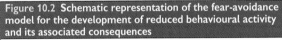

Table 10.1 Some of the major themes identified in qualitative analyses of the experience of chronic pain

- The struggle to feel that one's account of pain is believed by others, including health professionals
- The challenge of retaining a view of the self as a competent person
- Social distancing from others
- A distanced and changed view of ones physical self
- That ones current self is not ones 'real self'—the idea that the real self is suspended at some point in the past

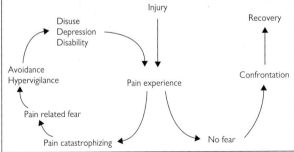

Figure 10.2 Schematic representation of the fear-avoidance model for the development of reduced behavioural activity and its associated consequences

Injury

Disuse
Depression
Disability

Recovery

Avoidance
Hypervigilance

Pain experience

Confrontation

Pain related fear

Pain catastrophizing

No fear

Figure 10.2 At the core of this model is the mediating role of catastrophic appraisals and fear that movement will result in significant harm. After Vlaeyen & Linton (2000).

10.5 **Effectiveness of psychological treatments**

The current psychological approach pain management—cognitive behaviour therapy—has been informed by development in the general field of psychotherapy over the past 40 years. As a result, treatments are multimodal and incorporate a range of behavioural and cognitive interventions that are presented to the patient during treatment sessions. Many treatment programmes are delivered in a group setting, which not only has economic advantages, but also enables the additional psychological characteristics of groups to be used to facilitate change. In addition to specific interventions such as pacing and shaping of behavioural change, central features of CBT are the attempt to engage patients in a collaborative partnership and the provision of education about chronic pain. Nevertheless, psychological treatment for chronic pain is characterized by considerable heterogeneity in several domains.

- The components therapy of included in treatment may vary between treatment centres and trials
- There is diagnostic variation between patients. Nevertheless, there is not much evidence to suggest that particular diagnostic categories are associated with specific psychological profiles. Rather it seems that empirically derived psychological profiles are independent of medical diagnosis, suggesting that it is the experience of chronic pain *per se* rather than diagnosis that is important
- There is variation in the measures used to assess outcomes. This reflects the fact that the aim of psychological treatments is to change a person's experience of pain and their ability to cope with it despite the persistence of pain. Pain reduction is often *not* a major focus of treatment.

There are now more than 40 RCTs of psychological treatments for chronic pain and despite the marked heterogeneity it is possible to draw some general conclusions about the efficacy of psychological treatments. A meta-analysis of trials published up to 1997 concluded that there was evidence of absolute efficacy, i.e. treatment is more effective than no treatment (waiting list control) for a range of outcomes and also that there was evidence of relative efficacy for several outcome domains when CBT was compared with other bona fide active treatments (Figure 10.3). These results have largely been supported by more recent meta-analyses for specific disorders (Hoffman *et al.*, 2007); nevertheless, a further analysis incorporating newer trials and more sophisticated statistical modelling is awaited.

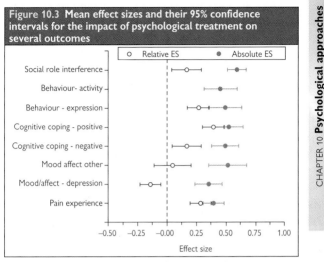

Figure 10.3 Mean effect sizes and their 95% confidence intervals for the impact of psychological treatment on several outcomes

The solid circles (•) indicate estimates of absolute efficacy (psychological treatment vs. no treatment): open circles (○) indicate estimates of relative effect sizes (psychological treatment vs. other bona fide treatment). Data from Morley et al. (1999).

10.6 **Conclusions**

The psychology of chronic pain is a complex and developing field. This chapter has briefly outlined a simple schematic framework into which the main issues can be accommodated.

Key references

Aldrich S, Eccleston C, Crombez G (2000). Worrying about chronic pain: vigilance to threat and misdirected problem solving. *Behav. Res. Ther.* **38**: 457–70.

Chibnall JT, Tait RC (1994). The Pain Disability Index: factor structure and normative data. *Arch. Phys. Med. Rehabil.* **75**: 1082–6.

Contrada RJ, Ashmore RD (eds) (1999). *Self, Social Identity, and Physical Health: Interdisciplinary Explorations.* Oxford University Press, New York.

Crombez G (2006). Hypervigilance and attention to pain: experimental and clinical evidence. In H Flor, E Kalso, JO Dostrovsky (eds), *Proceedings of the 11th World Congress on Pain* (pp. 515–28). IASP, Seattle.

Crombez G, Vlaeyen JW, Heuts PH, Lysens R (1999). Pain-related fear is more disabling than pain itself: evidence on the role of pain-related fear in chronic back pain disability. *Pain* **80** (1–2): 329–39.

De Vlieger P, Bussche EV, Eccleston C, Crombez G (2006). Finding a solution to the problem of pain: conceptual formulation and the development of the Pain Solutions Questionnaire (PaSol). *Pain* **123** (3): 285–93.

Eccleston C, Crombez G (1999). Pain demands attention: a cognitive-affective model of the interruptive function of pain. *Psychol. Bull.* **125** (3): 356–66.

Follick MJ, Smith TW, Ahern DK (1985). The sickness impact profile: a global measure of disability in chronic low back pain. *Pain* **21** (1): 67–76.

Grisart JM, Van der Linden M (2001). Conscious and automatic uses of memory in chronic pain patients. *Pain* **94** (3): 305–13.

Grisart J, Van der Linden M, Masquelier E (2002). Controlled processes and automaticity in memory functioning in fibromyalgia patients: relation with emotional distress and hypervigilance. *J. Clin. Exp. Neuropsychol.* **24** (8): 994–1009.

Hasenbring MI, Plaas H, Fischbein B, Willburger R (2006). The relationship between activity and pain in patients 6 months after lumbar disc surgery: do pain-related coping modes act as moderator variables? *Eur. J. Pain* **10** (8): 701–9.

Hoffman BM, Papas RK, Chatkoff DK, Kerns RD (2007). Meta-analysis of psychological interventions for chronic low back pain. *Health Psychol.* **26** (1): 1–9.

Kotarba JA (1983). *Chronic Pain: Its Social Dimension*. Sage Publications Inc., Beverly Hills.

McCracken LM (2005). *Contextual Cognitive-Behavioral Therapy for Chronic Pain* (Vol. 33). IASP Press, Seattle.

McCracken LM, Carson JW, Eccleston C, Keefe FJ (2004). Acceptance and change in the context of chronic pain. *Pain* **109** (1–2): 4–7.

Morley S, Davies C, Barton S (2005). Possible selves in chronic pain: self-pain enmeshment, adjustment and acceptance. *Pain* **115** (1–2): 84–94.

Morley S, Eccleston C, Williams A. Systematic review and meta-analysis of randomized controlled trials of cognitive behaviour therapy and behaviour therapy for chronic pain in adults, excluding headache. Pain 1999; **80**: 1–13.

Osborn M, Smith JA (1998). The personal experience of chronic benign lower back pain: an interpretative phenomenological analysis. *Br. J. Health Psychol.* **3**: 65–83.

Pincus T, Morley S (2001). Cognitive processing bias in chronic pain: a review and integration. *Psychol. Bull.* **127**: 599–617.

Sanders SH (2002). Operant conditioning with chronic pain: back to basics. In DC Turk, RJ Gatchel (eds), *Psychological Approaches to Pain Management: A Practitioner's Handbook.* (2nd ed., pp. 128–37). Guilford Press, New York.

Vlaeyen J, de Jong J, Seiben J, Crombez G (2002). Graded exposure *in vivo* for pain-related fear. In DC Turk, RJ Gatchel (eds), *Psychological Approaches to Pain Management: A Practitioner's Handbook* (2nd ed., pp. 210–33). Guilford Press, New York.

Vlaeyen JW, Linton SJ (2000). Fear-avoidance and its consequences in chronic musculoskeletal pain: a state of the art. *Pain* **85** (3): 317–32.

Vlaeyen JWS, Morley S (2004). Active despite pain: the putative role of stop-rules and current mood. *Pain* **110** (3): 512–16.

Index

A

acceptance and commitment therapy (ACT) 134–35
acetaminophen see paracetamol
acupuncture
  biological rationale/ plausibility 124–25
  clinical effectiveness 125–26
  contraindications/ precautions 125
  point selection 125
  technique 124
  timing/dosage 125
acute pain, definition of 2
AL-TENS (acupuncture-like TENS) 120
alcohol
  drug interactions 66
  neurolysis 95, 104
alfentanil 32, 93
allodynia, definition of 3
amitriptyline 63, 64, 67
amputation 7
analgesic ladder, WHO 31
analgesics, simple
  key points 15
  non-steroidal anti-inflammatory drugs (NSAIDs) 15, 17–23
  opioids, and synergistic analgesia 15
  paracetamol 15–17
anti-arrhythmics 66
  see also lidocaine; mexiletine
anti-hypertensives 78
anticoagulants 23
antidepressants
  amitriptyline 63
  duloxetine 27, 28, 41, 63, 67–8
  key points 63
  selective serotonin re-uptake inhibitors (SSRIs) 63, 65
  venlafaxine 67
  see also tricyclic antidepressants
antiepileptics 66, 67
  carbamazepine 53, 54–6
  clonazepam 53, 55, 61
  gabapentin 53, 56–8
  key points 53
  lamotrigine 53, 61

  levetiracetam 61
  mechanism of 53
  phenytoin 48, 53, 61, 78
  pregabalin 53, 58–61
  sodium valproate 53
  tiagabine 61
  topiramate 53, 61
antipsychotics 66
antiretrovirals 48
arthritis 4
aspirin 18, 20, 21, 22, 23, 45, 77, 78, 98

B

back pain
  epidemiology and impact of 4–5
  McKenzie therapy 127
  psychological factors 5–6
baclofen 82
balneotherapy 127
behavioural analysis 133–34
benzodiazepine 81
bisphosphonates
  administration 73
  adverse effects 72
  contraindications/precautions 72
  drug interactions 73
  pharmacology 72
botulinium toxin 98
breakthrough pain, definition of 3
bretylium 97
bupivacaine 75, 95
  coeliac plexus block 102, 104
  stellate ganglion block 100
buprenorphine 32
  administration 47
  adverse effects 46–7
  contraindications/precautions 46
  drug interactions 47
  pharmacology 46
  stellate ganglion block 100

C

calcitonin 82
cancer-related pain management 9
capsaican, topical 85–6
carbamazepine 53
  administration 56
  adverse effects 55

  contraindications/ precautions 54–5
  drug interactions 28, 47, 48, 55–6, 78, 81
  pharmacology 54
  special considerations 55
  trigeminal neuralgia 8
celecoxib 19, 23
central pain 7
central post-stroke pain (CPSP) 7
cervical facet joint injections (CFJI) 105
cervical nerve root block 108
children, pain in 10
chronic pain
  aetiology 6–9
  definition of 2
  epidemiology 4–6
  family involvement 5–6
  impact 4–6
  psychological factors 5–6
  risk factors 6
'chronic pain patient' 1
citalopram 28, 65
clodronate 72
clomipramine 64
clonazepam 53, 55, 61
clonidine 66, 87
  administration 73, 74–5
  adverse effects 74
  contraindications/ precautions 74
  drug interactions 74
  pharmacology 74
clopidogrel 98
co-proxamol 41
codeine 31
  administration 41
  adverse effects 41
  contraindications/ precautions 41
  drug interactions 41
  pharmacology 40
coeliac plexus block
  benefits/repeatability 104
  contraindications 103
  end points 103
  indications 102–3
  special points 103
  technique 103–4
cognitive-affective model of pain 132
cognitive behaviour therapy (CBT) 136
cognitive mediation hypothesis 134

cognitive therapy 134
complex regional pain
  syndrome (CRPS) 7–8
corticosteroids 22, 55
  administration 78
  adverse effects 77
  approximate equivalent
    anti-inflammatory
    doses 76
  contraindications/
    precautions 75–6
  depot steroids 95, 104
  drug interactions 77
  myofascial trigger point
    (MTP) injections 98
  pharmacology 75
  steroid withdrawal 76
COX-1 16, 18, 19, 21
COX-2 15, 18, 19, 20, 21,
  22, 23
COX-3 16, 19
cryotherapy 95
CT scan 95
ciclosporin 22, 23, 55
CYP1A2 70, 71
CYP3A4 26, 28, 55, 70, 71,
  80, 81
CYP2B6 26
CYP2C9 55
CYP2D6 26, 27, 70, 71

D

deep brain stimulation
  (DBS) 116–17
depot steroids
  nerve blocking solutions
    95
  pancreatitis 104
desipramine 65
dexamethasone 76
dextropropoxyphene 41
diamorphine 36, 40
diazepam 81
diclofenac 19
digoxin 78
dihydrocodeine 31
disability
  chronic pain 5–6
  WHO definition of 2
doloexetine 64
doxepin 88
drug interactions, elderly
  patients 10
duloxetine 27, 28, 41, 63,
  67–8

E

efavirenz 48
elderly, pain in 10
epidural blockade 110–11
epiduroscopy 111–12
erythromycin 48
etodolac 19

evidence-based clinical
  practice guidelines 128
extracorporeal shock wave
  therapy (ESWT) 127

F

facial pain 8
failed back surgery
  syndrome (FBSS) 5
fear-avoidance model of
  pain 134, 135
fentanyl 32, 36
  administration 42–4
  adverse effects 42
  contraindications/
    precautions 42
  drug interactions 42
  transdermal fentanyl patch
    42–3
flecainide 69
fluconazole 23
fluoroscopy 95
fluoxetine 27, 28, 41, 48,
  63, 65, 67

G

gabapentin 53, 87
  administration 58
  adverse effects 57
  contraindications/
    precautions 57
  dosage adjustments, renal
    function 58, 59
  dosage schedules 58
  drug interactions 57
  pharmacology 56–7
ganglion impar block 105
guanethidine 97

H

haloperidol 27, 41, 56
handicap, WHO definition
  of 2
headaches 8, 110
heroin see diamorphine
herpes zoster 8–9
HIV-related pain 8
Horner's syndrome 100
hydromorphone 32, 44, 114
hyperalgesia, definition of 3
hyperpathia, definition of 3
hypogastric block 105
hyponatraemia 55

I

iatrogenic neuropathic pain
  7
ibandronic acid 72, 73
ibuprofen 20, 22
imipramine 64
incident pain, definition of 3

infection 8–9
inorganic pyrophosphae
  71–2
interferential therapy (IFT)
  120
interspinous process
  distractor (X-STOP) 113
interventional anaesthetic
  techniques
  central blocks 110–16
  coeliac plexus block
    102–4
  ganglion impar block 105
  general principles 93–5
  headaches, nerve blocks
    for 110
  hypogastric block 105
  intravenous techniques
    96–7
  joint injections 105–7
  key points 93
  local anaesthetic injections
    97–9
  lumbar sympathetic block
    101–2
  nerve blocking solutions
    94–5
  nerve stimulators 94
  peripheral nerve blocks
    108–10
  renal nerve block 102,
    104–5
  sedation 94
  stellate ganglion block
    100–1
  sympathetic blocks
    99–100
  thoracic sympathectomy
    101
  ultrasound 95
intra-articular injection 107
intracellular cyclic adenosine
  monophosphate (cAMP)
  32
intradiscal electrothermal
  therapy (IDET) 112–13
intrathecal drug delivery
  (ITDD)
  complications 115
  contraindications 114
  evidence 115
  indications 114
  pre-procedure
    considerations 114
  special points 115
  technique 114

J

joint injections
  cervical facet joint
    injections (CFJI) 105
  intra-articular injection
    107
  lumbar facet joint
    injections (LFJI) 106

medial branch nerve
    denervation of facet
    joints 106–7
sacroiliac joint injections
    (SIJI) 106
thoracic facet joint
    injections (TFJI) 105

K

ketamine
    administration 81
    adverse effects 80–1
    burst ketamine therapy
        81, 82
    contraindications/
        precautions 80
    dosing regimes 81–2
    drug interactions 81
    intravenous techniques
        96
    pharmacology 79–80
    topical 88
ketoconazole 47
ketorolac 23
kyphoplasty 113

L

lamotrigine 53, 61
levetiracetam 61
levo-bupivacaine 95, 100
levomepromazine 27, 41, 74
lidocaine
    administration 71
    adverse effects 69–70
    coeliac plexus block 104
    contraindications/
        precautions 69
    drug interactions 71
    intravenous techniques 96
    local anaesthetics 95
    lumbar sympathetic block
        101
    pharmacology 69–70
    stellate ganglion block
        100
    topical and intravenous 69
    topical lidocaine 5%
        plaster 83–5
life-limiting pain 9
lithium 23
local anaesthetic injections
    97–9
lofepramine 65
lower level laser therapy
    (LLLT) 127
lumbar facet joint injections
    (LFJI) 106
lumbar nerve root block
    109
lumbar sympathetic block
    benefits/repeatability 102
    complications/side effects
        101–2
    technique 101

M

McKenzie therapy 127
medial branch nerve
    denervation of facet
    joints 106–7
meloxicam 19
methadone 56
    administration 48–9
    adverse effects 48
    contraindications/
        precautions 48
    drug interactions 48
    pharmacology 48
    titration methods,
        suggested 49
    transdermal patch initiation
        and titration 47
methionine 17
methotrexate 23
methylprednisolone 76
metoclopramide 28
metrizamide 95
mexiletine
    adverse effects 69–70
    contraindications/
        precautions 69
    drug interactions 71
    pharmacology 69–70
microcurrent stimulation
    120
midazolam 81, 93
migraine 8
mirtazapine 56, 63
misoprostol 23, 77
monoamine oxidase (MAO)
    27, 28, 39, 63, 66
morphine 31, 36
administration 37, 38, 39–40
    adverse effects 39
    contraindica-
        tions/precautions 38
    drug interactions 39–40
    as gold standard 37
    initiation and titration 35
    intrathecal drug delivery
        (ITDD) 114
    pharmacology 37–8
    stellate ganglion block
        100
    transdermal fentanyl patch
        conversion 43
morphine 3-glucuronide
    (M3G) 37, 38
morphine 6-glucuronide
    (M6G) 37, 38
motor cortex stimulation
    (MCS) 116–17
musculoskeletal pain 6
myeloscopy 111–12
myofascial trigger point
    (MTP) injections
    benefits 99
    contraindications 98
    myofascial versus nerve
        root pain 97

repeatability 99
side effects 99
special points 97–8
technique 98

N

N-acteyl-p-benzoquinimine
    (NAPQI) 16
N-methyl-D-aspartate
    (NMDA) receptors
    79–80, 81, 96
naloxone 32
naproxen 19
nefopam 82
nelfinavir 48
nerve blocking solutions
    depot steroids 95
    local anaesthetics 95
    neurolysis 95
nerve stimulators 94
neurolytic coeliac plexus
    block (NCPB) 104
neuropathic pain
    definition of 2–3
    diagnosis of 3
    prevalence of 3
    treatment of 3
nociceptive pain, definition
    of 2
non-pharmacological
    approaches
    acupuncture 124–26
    key points 119
    physiotherapy approaches
        126–28
    transcutaneous electrical
        nerve stimulation
        (TENS) 119–24
non-steroidal anti-
    inflammatory drugs
    (NSAIDs) 15
    absorption 19
    administration 23, 87
    adverse effects 21, 87
    contraindications/
        precautions 19–20, 87
    drug interactions 22, 77,
        78
    GI ulcers/perforation 19
    pharmacology 18–19, 86
    risk factors 21– 22
    topical analgesia 86–7
    use/actions 17
noradrenaline 64, 65, 67
norketamine 80
nortriptyline 64

O

oestrogens 56
ondansetron 28
operant learning theory
    133–34
opioids 66

addiction 33, 34
administration routes 36–7
benefits and abuse of 31
buccal administration 36–7
buprenorphine 46–7
cancer pain management 31
codeine 40–1
consideration of use of 33–4
definition of 31–2
dependence 33
diamorphine 40
fentanyl 41–4
hydromorphone 32, 44, 114
initiation and titration 35
intravenous techniques 96
key points 31
long-term opioids therapy, risks of 34
methadone 47–9
morphine 35, 37–40
non-cancer pain 33–5
opioid therapy, aim of 33
oral route 36
oxycodone 45–6
parenteral opioids 37
persistent pain management 31
pharmacology of 32
prescribing recommendations 34–5
rectal route 36
sedation effect 35
side effects 34, 35
spinal opioids 37
sublingual route 37
tolerance 33
topical 87–8
transdermal route 36
'weak' and 'strong' 31
withdrawal effects 33
oral transmucosal fentanyl citrate (OTFC) 36
oxycodone 32
administration 45–6
contraindications/precautions 45
drug interactions 45
pharmacology 45

P

pain, biopsychosocial model of 126
pain causation 1
Pain Disability Index 133
pain management
administration route 12
assessment 1
community-based services 11

multidisciplinary team approach 11
nerve block 12
neuromodulation 12
palliative care 11
patient/carer education 12–13
pharmacological therapies 11–12
physical interventions 12
primary care services 11
rehabilitation 12
secondary care services 11
specialist pain management 11
treatments, range of 11–13
Pain®Gone pens 120
pancreatitis 9, 104
Papaver somniferum (poppy) 31
paracetamol
administration/dosage 17
adverse effects 16
contraindications/precautions 16
drug interactions 17
pharmacology 15–16
toxicity 16–17
see also co-proxamol
paroxetine 27, 28, 41, 65
pentoxifylline 22
peripheral nerve blocks
cervical nerve root block 108
lumbar nerve root block 109
sacral nerve root block (SNRB) 109–10
selective nerve root blocks 108
thoracic nerve root block 108–9
peripheral nerve pain 7–8
pethidine 32, 41
phantom limb pain 7
phantom sensation 7
phenacetin 15
phencyclidine 78
phenol 95, 104
phentolamine 96–7
phenytoin 48, 53, 61, 78, 97
physiotherapy approaches
balneotherapy 127
clinical effectiveness 126–28
evidence-based clinical practice guidelines 128
exercise 126–27
extracorporeal shock wave therapy (ESWT) 127
lower level laser therapy (LLLT) 127

manipulation/mobilization 126
massage 126
pain, biopsychosocial model of 126
spa therapy 127
supervised physiotherapy 127
traction 127
ultrasound 127
piroxicam 19, 22
post-herpetic neuralgia (PHN) 8–9
post-surgical pain 7
post-traumatic pain
amputation 7
brachial plexus avulsion 6
vertebral crush fractures 7
prednisolone 76
pregabalin 53
administration 60–1
adverse effects 60
contraindications/precautions 59–60
dosage adjustments, renal function 60, 61
drug interactions 60
pharmacology 59
progestogens 56
propofol 93
prostaglandin biosynthesis 18–19, 21
prostaglandin E$_2$ production 83
psychological approaches
chronic pain, impact of 131–32
cognitive-affective model of pain 132
cognitive behaviour therapy (CBT) 136
cognitive mediation hypothesis 134
cognitive therapy 134
effectiveness of 136–37
fear-avoidance model of pain 134, 135
identity, impact of pain on 134–35
individual differences 132, 133
interference, from pain 133–34
interruption, caused by pain 132–33
key points 131
operant learning theory 133–34
pain intensity 133
performance, reduction in 133–34
primary task paradigm 132
psychological cascade schema 132

Q

quinolone antibiotics 23

R

radiofrequency lesioning 95
regional sympathetic
   blockade 97
remifentanil 94, 96
renal nerve block 102,
   104–5
rifampicin 67
ritonavir 48

S

sacral nerve root block
   (SNRB) 109–10
sacroiliac joint injections
   (SIJI) 106
selective nerve root blocks
   108
selective serotonin
   re-uptake inhibitors
   (SSRIs) 63, 65
serotonin 24, 26, 64, 65
serotonin and noradrenaline
   re-uptake inhibitors
   (SNRIs) 63, 65
serotonin syndrome 28, 45,
   66
serotoninergic (5-HT)
   neurotransmitter system
   16
sertraline 63
Sickness Impact Profile 133
sodium valproate 53
spa therapy 127
spinal cord stimulation
   (SCS)
   contraindications 115
   indications 116
   side effects 116
   techniques 115–16
   vascular pain 9
spinoscopy 111–12
spontaneous pain, definition
   of 3
stellate ganglion block
   benefits/repeatability 101

complications/side effects
   100–1
end points 100
technique 100–1
steroids see corticosteroids
stump pain 7
sympathetic blocks
   complications/side effects
   100
   contraindications 99
   indications 99
symptoms 1

T

thoracic facet joint
   injections (TFJI) 105
thoracic nerve root block
   108–9
thoracic sympathectomy
   101
tiagabine 61
topical analgesia
   advantages of 83
   capsaicin 85–6
   doxepin 88
   ketamine 88
   lidocaine 5% plaster 83–5
   nonsteroidal anti-
      inflammatory drugs
      (NSAIDs) 86–7
   opioids 87–8
   prostglandin E_2 production
      83
topiramate 53, 61
traction 127
tramadol 67
   administration 28
   adverse effects 27
   clinical efficacy 25
   contraindications/
      precautions 27
   drug interactions 25–6,
      27–8
   foetal development 27
   key points 25
   pharmacology 25–7
transcutaneous electrical
   nerve stimulation
   (TENS) 12
   biological rationale/
      plausibility 120, 121

clinical effectiveness 123
contraindications/
   precautions 121, 123
electrical characteristics
   121, 123
electrode position
   120–21, 122
technique 119–20
timing/dosage 121
transcutaneous spinal
   electroanalgesia (TSE)
   120
transdermal fentanyl patch
   42–3
transient receptor potential
   V1 ion channel (TRPV1)
   83, 85
tricyclic antidepressants 28,
   39, 63
   administration 64, 67
   adverse effects 66–7
   contraindications/
      precautions 64–6
   drug interactions 66–7
   pharmacology 64, 65
   secondary and tertiary
      64
   see also antidepressants
trigeminal neuralgia 8

U

ultrasound 95, 127

V

vascular pain 9
venlafaxine 28, 63, 65, 67
vertebroplasty 113
visceral pain 9
vulnerable groups, and pain
   management 10–11

W

warfarin 17, 67

Z

ziconotide 82, 114
zoledronic acid 72, 73